**DATE DUE**

the**facts**

# Insomnia and other adult sleep problems

# → also available in the**facts** series

# the**facts**

# Insomnia and other adult sleep problems
## PROFESSOR GREGORY STORES

616.8498
S 884

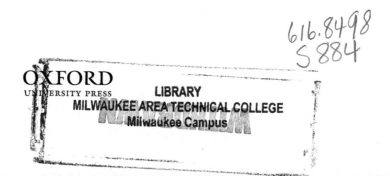

OXFORD
UNIVERSITY PRESS

LIBRARY
MILWAUKEE AREA TECHNICAL COLLEGE
Milwaukee Campus

# OXFORD

UNIVERSITY PRESS

Great Clarendon Street, Oxford OX2 6DP

Oxford University Press is a department of the University of Oxford.
It furthers the University's objective of excellence in research, scholarship,
and education by publishing worldwide in

Oxford New York

Auckland Cape Town Dar es Salaam Hong Kong Karachi
Kuala Lumpur Madrid Melbourne Mexico City Nairobi
New Delhi Shanghai Taipei Toronto

With offices in

Argentina Austria Brazil Chile Czech Republic France Greece
Guatemala Hungary Italy Japan Poland Portugal Singapore
South Korea Switzerland Thailand Turkey Ukraine Vietnam

Oxford is a registered trade mark of Oxford University Press
in the UK and in certain other countries

Published in the United States
by Oxford University Press Inc., New York

© Oxford University Press, 2009

The moral rights of the authors have been asserted
Database right Oxford University Press (maker)

First published 2009

All rights reserved. No part of this publication may be reproduced,
stored in a retrieval system, or transmitted, in any form or by any means,
without the prior permission in writing of Oxford University Press,
or as expressly permitted by law, or under terms agreed with the appropriate
reprographics rights organization. Enquiries concerning reproduction
outside the scope of the above should be sent to the Rights Department,
Oxford University Press, at the address above

You must not circulate this book in any other binding or cover
and you must impose this same condition on any acquirer

British Library Cataloguing in Publication Data

Data available

Library of Congress Cataloging in Publication Data
Stores, Gregory.
  Insomnia and other adult sleep problems / Gregory Stores.
    p. cm. -- (The facts)
  Includes index.
  ISBN 978-0-19-956083-7
  1. Insomnia. 2. Sleep disorders. I. Title.
  RC548.S76 2009
  616.8e'4982--dc22

                                                          2008041665

Typeset in Plantin
by Cepha Imaging Pvt. Ltd., Bangalore, India
Printed in China
through
Asia Pacific Offset

ISBN 978–0–19–956083–7 (Pbk.)

1 3 5 7 9 10 8 6 4 2

While every effort has been made to ensure that the contents of this book are as complete,
accurate, and up-to-date as possible at the date of writing, Oxford University Press is not able
to give any guarantee or assurance that such is the case. Readers are urged to take appropriately
qualified medical advice in all cases. The information in this book is intended to be useful to
the general reader, but should not be used as a means of self-diagnosis or for the prescription of
medication. The author and the publishers do not accept responsibility or legal liability for any
errors in the text or for the misuse or misapplication of material in this book.

# Foreword

Insomnia and other sleep problems comprise a common but generally poorly managed group of disorders. It is important to have some idea of what should be regarded as normal sleep, in terms of both duration and quality. There is great variation and what is normal for one individual is not for another. Reference is made to 6–8 hours of sleep as normal for adults, but many people—some well known, such as Margaret Thatcher and Winston Churchill—can function with much less.

For the general public, disturbed sleep is often not something they like to bother their doctor with, and yet, if persistent, it can have a devastating effect on their lives and that of their family. Health professionals, on the whole, are not always familiar with the large number of causes of disturbed sleep. Reference may be made to sleep disturbance as a symptom of certain specific diseases, but it is not often considered a topic in its own right. One hears, all too often, of a visit to the doctor to discuss insomnia resulting in a prescription for sleeping tablets. While on occasions this may be appropriate, generally the prescription pad is reached for too quickly. It is perfectly understandable for a busy GP with a shortage of time not to enquire more deeply into the precise nature of the problem, but it may also be a result of insufficient knowledge of the many causes of and reasons for sleep difficulties.

This book, with its reader-friendly style and layout, will help the general public to recognize the type of sleep problem that may be affecting them, or a close relative or friend, and to realize that help is available, and to show them how to find that help.

T.P. Dudeney MB BS MRCGP

General Practitioner

# Contents

# 1

# Introduction

## ➡ Key points

◆ Sleep is an essential part of human existence.

◆ Disturbed sleep (which is common) can have various serious consequences, especially concerning mood, behaviour, performance at work or at school, and social relationships.

◆ It is essential, therefore, that people seek help for their sleep problems and that effective treatment is provided.

## Differing attitudes to sleep

Attitudes to sleep vary significantly from one person to another. Some see it as an enjoyable experience and even a relief from daytime pressures and cares—a view expressed poetically by Sir Philip Sidney (1554–1586):

> Come, Sleep! O Sleep, the certain knot of peace,
> The baiting-place of wit, the balm of woe,
> The poor man's wealth, the prisoner's release,
> Th'indifferent judge between the high and low.
> *Astrophel and Stella* (*Certain Sonnets*, Sonnet **XXXIIX**)

On the other hand, those who sleep badly can regard the night as a distressing time, sometimes even to be dreaded, partly because of their inability to sleep but also because things can generally seem much worse at night than during the day. Literature again illustrates the point in Shakespeare's *Macbeth*:

> Good things of day begin to droop and drowse,
> Whiles night's black agents to their preys do rouse.
> *Macbeth*, III, ii, 45

If you sleep well and enjoy sleep, you might not mind that much of your life is spent asleep—on average 24 years, or even more allowing for the greater proportion of time that we sleep as children. However, if you are a poor sleeper, you are more likely to regret the proportion of your life that you spend sleeping—or trying to do so. Even if you have no trouble sleeping, you might resent the need to 'waste' time that might otherwise be used for more interesting and productive activities.

Some species of animal do not suffer this disadvantage: while one half of their brain (or cerebral hemisphere) is asleep, the other half remains awake! Examples of this so-called 'unihemispheric sleep' include certain types of dolphin and porpoise.

Sadly (at least for those frustrated by having to sleep), we show no capacity for this type of sleep. Instead, we need to sleep solidly and completely in order to function at our best during the day. Unfortunately, about a third or more of people of all ages have problems with their sleep, and many do not seek help, even though their poor sleep seriously affects their lives.

## Effects of poor sleep

You may already know from personal experience that persistent loss of sleep or disturbed sleep can cause all sorts of problems. Most people become tired, irritable, and out of sorts. Coping with everyday challenges or stresses becomes more difficult, causing upset, depression, and even aggression—and this affects family and friends. Children do less well at school and adults have difficulty doing their job properly, especially if it requires sustained concentration and effort.

Accidents at work or while driving are often caused by lack of sleep. Some major disasters, such as the Exxon Valdez oil tanker spillage and the explosion of the space shuttle Challenger in 1986, have been attributed to sleep disturbance in key personnel.

It has been estimated that the effects of sleep problems cost the USA many billions of dollars a year. It is likely that the economic consequences are similar in the UK and elsewhere.

For these various reasons, much more attention should be paid to the importance of sleeping well. However, in order to prevent or treat sleep problems, doctors and other professionals also need to know more about sleep and its disorders.

## Personal awareness of sleep disorders

Most people need to know more about the nature and importance of sleep to recognize in themselves and others the signs of unsatisfactory sleep and to know what they can do to help themselves and how best to obtain help.

It is particularly important that everyone should consider sleep a very important part of their lives and should ask for help at an early stage if they think that they (or someone close to them) have a sleep problem.

At present, comparatively few people seek help, even for serious sleep problems. For example, only about 10% of adults whose breathing is interrupted during sleep (see obstructive sleep apnoea, Chapter 9) seek help from their doctors, even though, as discussed later in the book, the condition results in poor-quality sleep and often severe daytime problems.

## Professional awareness of sleep disorders

Surveys carried out in the UK and elsewhere have shown that usually very little time (if any) is given to sleep and its disorders in the training of medical students, family doctors, hospital specialists, and nurses. The same is true of psychologists, teachers, and others involved in the care of people from childhood to old age. For example, medical students are taught to ask only superficial questions about patients' sleep. Qualified doctors in the various specialties may well fail to enquire about sleep problems in their patients, whether adults or children.

Thus, it is no surprise that many significant sleep problems are not recognized (still less treated properly) and that they continue to affect people's lives unnecessarily, quite possibly for years on end.

## Almost all sleep problems can be treated

Overall, there is a vast number of people with significant sleep problems who are not receiving help, mainly because they do not realize that they have a serious but treatable condition. If more people recognized the importance of seeking help with their sleep problems at an early stage—and insisted on getting it—improvements in the education and training of doctors and others would be much more likely to happen. All concerned need to realize that, in fact, there is a wide variety of types of treatment that can be used effectively if sought and then provided.

# The purpose of this book

This book is intended mainly to help members of the general public to recognize the importance of sleep and to understand its disorders (including their recognition, importance, and treatment) in adults. Some professionals may also find it useful.

It should help you towards an understanding of the modern approach to sleep problems and encourage healthy sleep patterns in yourself and others close to you, as well as encouraging you to seek the right kind of help when needed. It is hoped that it will contribute to a greater general awareness of the topic.

Certain points about the book should be emphasized.

◆ The account it provides is only general in nature, without any attempt to go into detail. For this, it would be necessary to consult more technical books such as those described under Sources of further information in the Appendix.

◆ The later chapters presuppose that the earlier chapters have been read.

◆ To aid understanding of certain points or concepts, reference is made to other chapters elsewhere in the book.

◆ The case studies have been made anonymous to preserve confidentiality.

◆ In places, reference is made to 'he' or 'his', and not to the female gender, for the sake of brevity.

◆ Reference is made to the kind of sleep problems that affect children and adolescents only in relation to the effects on their parents' sleep. A companion book specifically about the sleep problems of children and adolescents is available in this *Facts* series (see Appendix).

◆ **This book is not intended to be a substitute for medical advice from your own doctor**.

# 2

# Why is sleep so important?

## ➜ Key points

- There are many harmful effects of not sleeping well.

- If you have insufficient sleep, you may feel tired and sleepy, weary, irritable, aggressive, or depressed. Young children can become overactive. Other family members are also likely to be affected.

- Poor concentration and memory problems may also result, impairing performance at work or at school.

- Persistently disturbed sleep can also affect basic bodily processes, potentially causing physical ill-health.

There have been various theories about the function of sleep. For example, some have emphasized its role in brain development and in learning and memory. No one theory accounts for all of the complexities of sleep in different species and at different ages.

What is clear is that sleep is essential for recovery and restoration. Sustained effort leads to tiredness, fatigue, and the need to sleep. If sleep is persistently disturbed, you will be affected psychologically and perhaps physically.

## Sleep debt

Loss of sleep or poor-quality (non-restorative) sleep leads to the build-up of a 'sleep debt'. This increases the pressure to sleep in order to pay off the debt when the next opportunity to sleep becomes available. Repeatedly disturbed sleep progressively builds up the size of the sleep debt. Fortunately, it takes far less time to pay off this debt than it takes to incur it. In other words, a relatively short period of sound sleep is sufficient to offset the immediate effects of sleep loss.

---

### ❌ Myth versus fact

❌ **Myth:** You can get used to having less sleep if you try.

❗ **Fact:** This is unlikely. What might happen is that you forget what it is like to be at your best, as it is almost certain that less sleep than usual will make you less well in yourself.

---

## Effects of sleep disturbance on mood and behaviour

On the psychological side, the main effects are often on mood. In adults, this usually takes the form of irritability, generally feeling out of sorts, or exhaustion. If sleep has been seriously disturbed for a long time, it can lead to feelings of depression.

The inability to cope with demands at home and work can lead to further complications, which may result in unreasonable and even aggressive behaviour towards others. These and other harmful effects of the sleep disturbance itself are likely to be made worse when people try to treat their sleep problem themselves.

For example, some people unwisely use alcohol in an attempt to help them get to sleep; others take stimulant substances (such as large amounts of coffee or even stimulant drugs) to combat sleepiness during the day. Even prescribed sleeping tablets may actually make sleep problems worse (see Chapter 8).

As well as adults, children and adolescents can also react to sleep disturbance in these ways without the real cause of their behaviour being recognized, so that other, mistaken explanations are given (see Chapter 12). The situation can be further complicated psychologically if they become upset because they are distressed by their sleep problem or if their sleep pattern leads to confrontation with their parents.

An important difference between adults and children is that, whereas in adults disturbed sleep generally causes sleepiness and a reduction in activity, young children in particular can become overactive and disruptive. Attention-deficit hyperactivity disorder (ADHD) can be the result of disturbed sleep rather than the cause.

# Effects on social relationships

If one person has a sleep problem, the whole family may be upset by it. If your sleep is persistently disturbed, you are less likely to function well as a parent or partner, irrespective of whether the disturbance is caused by your own sleep disorder or that of your partner or child.

Some studies have found that mothers of children with severe sleep difficulties (and, presumably as a consequence, inadequate sleep of their own) have more health problems than average, are less affectionate towards their children, and may even use more physical punishment than other mothers. Marital discord and separation have been attributed to children's sleep problems in some cases.

Fortunately, there is evidence that successful treatment of a child's sleep disorder can help to resolve problems within the family, although this does not seem to be widely known and, therefore, the help required is often not provided.

# Effects on abilities and performance

Many experiments on sleep-deprived individuals have consistently shown that attention (especially when it has to be maintained for long periods), memory, and other abilities are affected. Creativity and abstract thinking can be particularly vulnerable to sleep disturbance.

These effects depend on a number of factors, such as how much sleep you have lost, individual personality, and how hard you try to perform well. People can differ considerably in how much they are affected, but, generally speaking, repeated disturbance of sleep at night causes significant problems. It has been calculated that some people with persistent loss of sleep perform only a tenth as well in memory and concentration tasks as those who usually sleep well.

The results of such experiments are in keeping with evidence that people whose jobs interfere seriously with normal sleep patterns are liable to have more health problems and to function less well at work, including being prone to mistakes and accidents.

People who are at increased risk of such problems (see also Chapter 11) include:

- shift workers;

- airline personnel including pilots (especially on long-haul flights, which result in jet lag);

- train drivers; and

- hospital doctors working long hours, including at night when their sleep may repeatedly be disrupted.

Research has shown that sleep loss in children and adolescents has an effect on attention and other intellectual abilities similar to that seen in adults. Reports from different countries have shown that inadequate sleep in children and adolescents, caused by late bedtimes and sometimes early school starting times, is associated with daytime sleepiness and poor progress at school (see Chapters 7 and 9).

## Physical effects

Children who have obstructive sleep apnoea (OSA) from an early age—possibly from around 2 years of age—can suffer physical consequences. Some of them will be underweight, in contrast to adults with OSA who are more likely to be overweight. The reason why physical growth is affected in this way is that deep sleep (during which growth hormone is produced) is disrupted. Removal of the obstruction that is stopping a child from breathing properly usually improves sleep and allows him to start growing normally again.

Adults with OSA run a serious risk of developing high blood pressure and heart problems, and possibly of having a stroke.

Recently, it has become apparent that night-shift work (which upsets your circadian rhythms in various ways; see Chapter 11) is associated with such physical disorders as gastrointestinal problems, raised blood pressure, and even complications during pregnancy.

There is increasing interest in yet other ways in which sleep loss or disruption can have harmful effects on basic bodily processes, including the immune system, which helps fight off infection, and various endocrine disorders.

## The extent of harmful effects and prospects of help

These various effects may well be widespread in the community, affecting people of all ages. For example, the well-being and intellectual competence of many elderly people (who are particularly prone to sleep problems) might be improved if they could be helped to sleep better (see Chapter 11).

At any age, physical and psychiatric illnesses are often complicated by sleep disturbance. If sleep is improved, the ill person may be able to cope better.

There are also certain physical conditions, in which sleepiness is a significant symptom, that also have serious psychological effects, which can be alleviated if the underlying disorder is treated effectively.

OSA (see Chapter 9) is a good example. In this condition, breathing difficulties, usually involving loud snoring, severely impair the individual's quality of sleep (as well as that of their bed partner). This can result in severe underperformance and other psychological difficulties during the day. Effective treatment of these breathing difficulties can bring about striking improvements in the person's daytime well-being and abilities. Similar benefits can also be seen in children with OSA (usually caused by enlarged tonsils and adenoids) and in some children and adults with nocturnal asthma. The successful treatment of narcolepsy (see Chapter 9) can have a similarly good effect.

Those caring at home for elderly or chronically ill people (including those with dementia; see Chapter 11) with severely disturbed sleep often face serious problems of their own because their sleep is disturbed. Both carers, and those for whom they care, would benefit from more help with their sleep disturbance.

## Conclusion

Overall, it is obvious that sleep is essential to refresh our brains and for us to function well—both psychologically and physically. If we lose out on sleep over a long period, or obtain only poor-quality sleep (see Chapter 5), we cannot function properly. Therefore, it is important to make sure that we all regularly sleep long enough each night, and that our sleep is sound, to ensure that we are restored and able to feel well and function satisfactorily during the day. It is also important to take steps as soon as possible to help those whose sleep is already disturbed.

# 3

# What is sleep?

## ⮕ Key points

◆ There are two distinct types of sleep—non-rapid eye movement (NREM) and rapid eye movement (REM) sleep—a balance of which is needed to function well during the day. During the night, these two types of sleep alternate with each other.

◆ Probably everyone dreams but the purpose of dreaming is generally unclear.

◆ The pattern of wakefulness and sleep is controlled by an internal clock in the brain (the body clock).

◆ Your level of alertness varies within each 24 hours. The tendency to sleep is greatest in the early hours of the morning (corresponding to deep NREM sleep) and (although less so) in the early afternoon.

◆ People vary in the time of day when they are most alert: 'larks' in the morning and 'owls' in the evening. Most people show neither of these patterns.

◆ Daytime naps can make it difficult to get to sleep at bedtime if they are too long or too late in the day. Long naps can make you feel groggy afterwards.

Sleep has some features in common with other states of relative inactivity, such as coma or, in some species, hibernation. All of these states usually occur while lying down with little movement and reduced awareness of the environment to varying degrees. However, sleep is very different from the rest. For instance, a sleeping person can be woken fairly easily and sleep usually occurs naturally in every 24-hour period. Also, in sleep, there is not simply a reduction in brain and other bodily activities as occurs in coma or hibernation.

Sleep involves complicated biochemical changes and activation of pathways in various parts of the brain. These allow us to go to sleep and then wake up again, and also to switch repeatedly during the night between very different types of sleep.

# Types of sleep

There are two types of sleep: NREM and REM sleep.

Why there are two types of sleep is not clear. Humans share this feature with certain other species, especially other primates. After loss of sleep, deep NREM sleep tends to be made up first, followed by REM sleep, suggesting that deep sleep is more important for restoring brain function. On the other hand, the proportion of REM sleep is greater in early development, as if it is particularly important for brain development and learning. It is likely that a combination of both types of sleep is needed to function well and remain healthy.

## NREM sleep

NREM sleep makes up about 75% of adult sleep. It is divided into four levels of increasing depth, called stages. Each stage has its own characteristic type of brain activity, as recorded by an electroencephalogram or EEG. The eyes are relatively still, most muscles are only somewhat relaxed, and breathing and heart rate are steady.

Stages 1 and 2 are relatively light sleep without any slow EEG activity. When we are deeply asleep we are in stages 3 and 4. This level of NREM sleep is also called slow-wave sleep (SWS) because, at this level, our brain activity consists mainly of large slow waves. It is especially difficult to waken from this level of sleep. SWS occurs mainly in the first 3 hours of sleep (see Figure 3.1).

Sleepwalking and related arousal disorder episodes (see Chapter 10) arise from SWS. Only fragments of dreams occur in NREM sleep.

## REM sleep

REM, where most dreaming occurs, is seen mostly later in the night (see Figure 3.1). The proportion of REM sleep is greatest in very young children. It takes up at least 50% of sleep in newborns (more than this before birth), reducing to 20–25% by about 2 years of age, and then stays at something like this level throughout the rest of life.

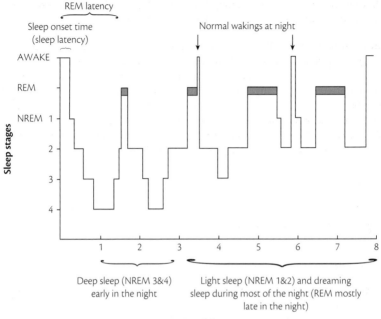

**Figure 3.1** Example of a hypnogram, showing the sequence of sleep stages

It is not obvious why REM sleep continues throughout our lives, although it is thought to have some part to play in memory. Adults deprived of REM sleep (either experimentally by waking them each time a period of REM sleep begins, or as a result of brain disorders affecting REM sleep mechanisms) are not necessarily affected in an obvious way, either intellectually or emotionally.

Your brain function is very active during REM sleep. This can be seen in an EEG and from studies that show that blood flow to the brain is increased compared with NREM sleep. Despite this, it is not usually possible for you to move much, if at all, during this type of sleep. For that reason, REM sleep is sometimes called 'paradoxical' sleep as the brain is active but the body is not.

Although in REM sleep your eyes move and the muscles involved in breathing continue to function, usually none of your other muscles can move, apart from perhaps a slight twitching. This is so even during dreams, which occur mainly during REM sleep (although not all REM sleep is taken up by dreaming). Some people have an abnormal ability to move during REM sleep and are thus able to act out their dreams. If the content of their dreams is violent, they will behave violently and may hurt themselves or others. This condition is called 'REM sleep behaviour disorder' (see Chapter 10).

In contrast to NREM sleep, your respiration and heart rate are somewhat irregular during REM sleep. Another feature is that, unlike in NREM sleep, men usually have penile erections (the equivalent in women is enlargement of the clitoris). These changes are not the result of erotic dreams because they can be observed in newborn babies. If difficulty achieving or maintaining an erection during sexual activity is caused by psychological factors, erections during REM sleep are still likely to occur. This is not so if the cause is physical, as might be the case in diabetes, for example.

## Dreaming

### ❌ Myth versus fact

❌ **Myth**: Dreaming is essential to be psychologically healthy.

❗ **Fact**: There is no convincing evidence for this. The reason why we dream is something of a mystery.

Dreams have intrigued people from ancient times, but the reason why we dream remains unclear. Most dreams occur in REM sleep later in the night or before waking, but dream-like experiences can also occur when drifting off to sleep. By waking people during REM sleep, research has shown that just about everybody has dreams. However, on waking normally, some people do not remember them when they wake up.

Sometimes the content of our dreams can be traced to recent experiences or preoccupations, but often it provides little insight into our daytime thoughts and feelings. An exception to this is recurrent upsetting dreams, which can have the same content each time. This can happen following bereavement or another traumatic experience.

Many people have occasional nightmares or frightening dreams (see Chapter 10) for no obvious reason. Recurrent nightmares suggest a significant emotional upset (as in post-traumatic stress disorder), which needs to be treated. Also, some medications can cause frequent nightmares.

Blind people dream but without any visual imagery if they have been blind from birth or since their early years.

# The pattern of overnight sleep

The way in which periods of NREM and REM sleep alternate with each other several times during the night is shown in Figure 3.1, which illustrates the pattern of overnight sleep that can be expected in a healthy young adult.

Ideally, about 20 minutes or less after settling in bed, drowsiness gives way to the lighter stages of NREM sleep and then, over the next 20 minutes or so, the deeper levels are reached. Around 40 minutes later, sleep lightens progressively until the first period of REM sleep occurs, lasting perhaps 10–15 minutes. After that, periods of NREM (with progressively lighter stages) and REM sleep alternate, each NREM–REM cycle lasting about 90 minutes.

Note that there is more deep NREM sleep in the first part of the night and progressively more REM sleep later on. For this reason, disturbances of sleep that arise in deep sleep (such as sleepwalking) usually occur in the first part of the night, but those linked to REM sleep (for example, nightmares) happen mainly later in the night.

Occasional brief waking during the night is normal at all ages, although it might not be remembered. A problem only arises if it is difficult to get back to sleep.

# The circadian body clock

Our need to sleep ('sleep drive') is determined by two influences, each of which involves different brain systems:

◆ the length of time that we have been awake; and

◆ our 'circadian body clock', which regulates when we sleep within each 24-hour period.

Many of our bodily functions fluctuate in cycles (or rhythms), which are regulated by our brain. The timing of these different rhythms ranges from minutes to days.

The timing of our sleep (but not how long we sleep) is regulated by what is called the 'circadian body clock', which is located in the suprachiasmatic nuclei (SCN) in the depths of the brain. Circadian (from *circa* meaning 'around' and *dies* meaning 'a day') refers to a daily rhythm that occurs about every 24 hours. Interestingly, left to its own devices (as it were), your body clock would organize your sleep–wake cycle to be slightly longer than 24 hours. This has implications for the development of jet lag, especially when travelling from west to east (see Chapter 11).

The circadian body clock also controls a number of other biological rhythms such as body temperature and cortisol, a hormone that is important in your response to stress. These rhythms are normally synchronized with each other—for example, body temperature falls during overnight sleep and is at its lowest levels in deep NREM sleep.

From an early age, the sleep–wake rhythm becomes linked in time with the night–day cycle ('entrainment'). This is achieved by means of various external time cues (zeitgebers, from a German word meaning literally 'time giver'). The main zeitgeber is the perception of variation in daylight, but other cues such as mealtimes and social activities are also important.

These other zeitgebers are important to blind people although the sleep–wake pattern of some blind people is still influenced by light during the day, even though they are not able to see it. It seems that this is because connections can still exist between the eye and the SCN without involving those parts of the brain on which perception of light depends.

## Melatonin

The SCN is influenced by a hormone called melatonin, which is produced mainly in a part of the brain called the pineal gland. Melatonin is secreted during darkness and is suppressed by exposure to bright light (usually sunlight)—hence its name, the 'hormone of darkness'. Thus, darkness promotes sleep and bright light encourages wakefulness.

In recent years, melatonin has achieved some popularity as a treatment for various sleep problems, but it does not always live up to this reputation, partly because of individual differences in response to taking it (see Chapter 11 for its possible value in various groups at special risk of sleep disorders).

## Disturbances in circadian rhythms

The various circadian rhythms can become out of step with each other ('desynchronized') with potentially serious effects. This desynchronization has been likened to all of the sections of an orchestra playing at different times, producing discord instead of harmony. This happens in certain sleep disorders such as those resulting from jet lag or night-shift work (see Chapter 11), in certain forms of depression, and possibly in the later years of life.

Although our natural sleep–wake period is about 24 hours, electric lighting in the evening tends to lengthen the awake phase artificially. Working late, or other activities late in the evening and into the early hours, further disrupts our natural sleep–wake rhythm. This can be a potent cause of inadequate sleep if you have to get up early for work or some other commitment (see, for example, delayed sleep-phase syndrome in Chapters 7 and 9).

# Variations in alertness and sleepiness within each 24 hours

In addition to circadian rhythms, there are other internal rhythms involving systems in the brain that affect our levels of alertness and sleepiness within each 24-hour period. These are called ultradian rhythms meaning 'occurring more than once each 24 hours'. Incidentally, a third kind of biological rhythm is where each period extends for longer than 24 hours; this is called an infradian rhythm, for example the menstrual cycle.

Our tendency to fall asleep is greatest in the early hours of the morning, corresponding to the slow-wave levels of NREM sleep and, to a lesser extent, we tend be sleepy in the early afternoon—the 'post-lunch dip'.

We are generally at our most alert in the evening before the onset of sleepiness. This period of highest alertness has been called the 'forbidden zone' because of the impossibility at that time of being able to get to sleep naturally. Parents' futile attempts to make their children go to sleep too early in the evening is one cause of bedtime problems. All things being equal, this period of maximal alertness is the best time to study.

Attempting to be active in the early hours of the morning, when our body clock is telling our brain that we should be deeply asleep, can cause serious problems. Night-shift workers (see Chapter 11) often have difficulty for this reason. Road accidents caused by a driver falling asleep at the wheel (see Chapter 11) are most common in the early hours of the morning and also (to a lesser extent) in the afternoon, corresponding to the periods when our infradian tendencies to sleep are greatest.

## Individual variations in infradian rhythms

Individuals vary in the precise timing of their peaks and troughs of alertness or sleepiness. Even from an early age, some people wake about 2 hours earlier than most other people and are especially alert and active in the morning. They then tire in the evening and are soon asleep. These are the 'morning types' or 'larks'.

In contrast, others tend to wake up 2 hours later than others and have particular difficulty getting up and functioning properly in the morning, but become at their most alert and active in the evening. They are called 'evening types' or 'owls'. About two-thirds of people are neither larks nor owls; they are described as 'indifferent types'.

These individual differences are referred to as 'chronotypes'. Along with other biological factors (such as age, gender, and general health), your chronotype will determine how readily you can adjust your circadian rhythms to a new sleep–wake cycle. For example, larks have the greatest difficulty coping with night-shift work.

## Napping

> ### ❌ Myth versus fact
>
> ❌ **Myth**: Daytime naps are useful if you have difficulty getting to sleep at night.
>
> ❗ **Fact**: Quite the opposite—napping during the day can make it more difficult to get to sleep.

Certain cultures make use of the post-lunch dip by taking a siesta each day and some adults in other countries are in the habit of taking a nap during the day. In these circumstances and, for example, to help avoid being sleepy when driving (see Chapter 11), there are certain important points to remember about napping.

- Naps are best taken in the early afternoon to coincide with the post-lunch dip. If taken later, they might make it difficult to get to sleep at bedtime.

- Each nap should be no longer than about 20 minutes to avoid going into SWS. As mentioned previously, it is difficult to waken from this depth of sleep and, after a longer nap, you are likely to be groggy and unable to function properly for a time ('sleep inertia').

- Napping at irregular times (including doing so only at weekends) can upset your body clock and make it difficult for you to sleep at night.

- Daytime naps should generally be taken only if you have no difficulty sleeping at night. Resist the temptation to sleep during the day because you feel tired as a result of not sleeping well at night, as this will make it even more difficult to get to sleep then.

# 4

# Changes in sleep with age

> ## ➲ Key points
>
> ◆ Very young children sleep most of the time, with a relatively high proportion spent in rapid eye movement (REM) sleep.
>
> ◆ Later (with the exception of adolescence), there is a gradual reduction in sleep requirements until early adult life when an average of 7–8 hours' sleep a night is needed to function well during the day. However, individual sleep requirements vary.
>
> ◆ These requirements remain fairly constant into old age when it can become difficult to maintain unbroken sleep.
>
> ◆ Adolescents often get less sleep than they need.

> ## ✖ Myth versus fact
>
> ✖ **Myth**: All adolescents are impossible to get up in the morning—it's just the way they are.
>
> ❗ **Fact**: It is true that adolescents often have a special need for sleep, but not all are difficult to rouse in the morning. Where this is a problem, there is likely to be a reason that can be put right.
>
> ✖ **Myth**: Old people don't need much sleep because they don't do much during the day.

> **❶ Fact**: Apart from the fact that the second half of this statement is often untrue, the amount of sleep needed to function at your best remains very much the same throughout adult life. There is likely to be a treatable cause if they do not sleep well.

The nature of our sleep, and how much sleep we need, changes considerably during the course of our lives. Table 4.1 shows the average amount of sleep needed at different ages. However, it is important to realize that, at any age, people differ somewhat from each other in this respect. As part of their biological make-up, a few can function perfectly well on less than the average; others may need more without having a sleep disorder.

The biggest changes occur during childhood (see Table 4.1). An understanding of children's sleep is important for adults because their own sleep may be affected as part of being a parent (see Chapter 11).

# Childhood

Children's sleep problems can disrupt their parents' sleep in various ways, which partly reflect the changes that occur in sleep during the course of early development.

## Babies

Studies of premature babies show that sleep begins well before birth. A fetus spends up to 20 hours a day asleep. This very high amount of sleep persists during infancy, with at least 50% of it taking the form of REM-type ('active') sleep. This compares with about 25% of REM sleep in early adult life, perhaps reducing somewhat in old age. Also, infants can pass directly into REM sleep when they fall asleep.

As their body clock has not yet developed properly, babies' sleep–wake patterns are generally so irregular that parents' sleep inevitably suffers because they have to wake repeatedly to feed or comfort their baby during the night. However, by 6 months (or even earlier), a full-term baby is biologically able to confine feeding to the daytime.

By the end of the first year, the average child still sleeps about 14 hours a day. Daytime naps should reduce to one or two and then to one by about 18 months before stopping altogether—usually by 3–4 years of age.

**Table 4.1** Usual sleep requirements over 24 hours at different ages (note that people differ somewhat in how much sleep they need)

| Age | Sleep requirements |
| --- | --- |
| Newborn, full-term baby. | 16–18 hours. |
| 1 year. | 14 hours. |
| 2 years. | 13 hours. |
| 4 years. | 11.5 hours. |
| 7 years. | 10.5 hours. |
| 10 years. | 9 hours. |
| Adolescence (after puberty). | 9 hours, possibly more (often less than this is obtained). |
| Late adolescence. | 8 hours. |
| Adulthood (including old age). | 7–8 hours. |

## Toddlers

Difficulties at bedtime and troublesome night-waking problems in toddlers are very common and are a serious concern to many parents. This is not only because of the stress caused at the time but also because of the effect on the parents' emotional state and general well-being of a recurrent lack of sleep (see Chapter 11).

## Older children

The sleep of older children (before puberty) is generally very efficient and sound. The sleep problems that often develop at this age (such as night-time fears or sleepwalking) seriously disrupt parents' sleep directly in only a small proportion of cases where the episodes are frequent.

The sleep of psychologically disturbed children (whatever the nature of the disturbance) is likely to be affected. Conversely, the main cause of some children's difficult behaviour is a sleep disorder. As mentioned earlier (see Chapter 2), attention-deficit hyperactivity disorder (ADHD) can be an example of this. Physical disorders causing pain or discomfort at night will disturb sleep at this and any other age.

## Adolescence

The progressive decline in the amount of sleep that children need as they get older tends to slow down or halt with the onset of puberty. At the same time, the body clock changes, increasing the tendency for a young person to be alert towards the end of the day at the time when previously they would have felt the need to sleep.

The combination of these biological changes and late-night social activities (recently including late-night use of mobile phones for texting) or studying late can shift the time of their period of sleep even later. The body clock can become set to the point where it is not possible to get to sleep until very late, no matter how hard the young person tries (see Chapter 7). The problems arising from this are that, because of these changes, many adolescents obtain less sleep at a time when they need more (see Chapter 11).

## Early adult life

By early adulthood, the amount of sleep that most people need to function satisfactorily has reduced to about 7–8 hours. Unfortunately, many adults seem to obtain less sleep than they need. This is largely because of lifestyle factors, including the demands of work or social activities. This sleep deprivation, or 'sleep debt', can cause the various psychological and physical problems discussed in Chapter 2. In these circumstances, getting more natural sleep each night is likely to make a person feel and perform better during the day. Even those who feel fine during the day may find that they feel even better if they alter their sleep habits so that they obtain at least an extra hour of sleep at night. This applies at all ages.

## Later in life

Elderly people do not necessarily need less sleep than when they were younger, but many achieve only poor-quality sleep partly because of the ageing process. 'Sleep efficiency' (the amount of time in bed actually asleep) is often reduced. They spend less time in deep non-rapid eye movement (NREM) sleep and their sleep tends to be more broken because of the brain's reduced ability to maintain sound sleep. Although it is normal at any age to wake occasionally during the night, this happens more frequently after the age of about 60.

In addition to these alterations in sleep quality, the body clock controlling circadian sleep and wakefulness changes again. In contrast to what happens in adolescence, elderly people tend to fall asleep earlier and wake up earlier (see Chapter 11). Also, if they nap a lot during the day (perhaps as a general lessening of daytime activity for whatever reason), this can cause further problems with night-time sleep. As people need only a certain amount of sleep in each 24 hours, taking daytime naps can mean that they are unable to sleep at night.

The combination of biological and altered lifestyle (for example, following retirement or bereavement), possibly complicated by various physical and psychological conditions that disturb sleep, increases the number of sleep complaints in later life (see Chapter 11). If a person suffers from dementia, sleep–wake patterns often become highly disrupted, creating considerable problems for carers (see Chapter 11).

# 5

# Signs of unsatisfactory sleep

## ➲ Key points

◆ Satisfactory sleep (i.e. of sufficient duration and quality) enables you to feel well and function at your best during the day.

◆ There are many possible signs that your sleep is unsatisfactory. These consist of difficulty getting up in the morning, and various problems during the day and at night.

◆ Some of the daytime effects of unsatisfactory sleep might be similar to those caused by other difficulties primarily of a physical or psychological nature. However, it is important that disturbed sleep is not overlooked as a cause of such problems.

◆ Equally, sleep disorders must not be misinterpreted as other clinical conditions.

## ❌ Myth versus fact

❌ **Myth**: The effects of not sleeping well are obvious to anyone, including yourself. You just feel tired.

❶ **Fact**: Actually, inadequate or poor-quality sleep can affect you in many different ways, both psychologically and physically. So much is this the case that often this explanation of your difficulties gets overlooked instead of being dealt with.

# What is satisfactory sleep?

Many people know they do not sleep well, although many do not ask for help and soldier on as best they can. Others are less aware that their sleep is unsatisfactory and that they could benefit if their sleep was improved. Ideally, a person's sleep at night should be both long enough (adequate sleep) and also of sufficiently good quality to restore them, so that they feel well and can function properly during the day.

Good-quality sleep means that sleep is sound and unbroken. In addition, sleep quality can be impaired (also called 'fragmented' sleep) by very brief arousals without you consciously waking up. This happens particularly in later life and in various sleep disorders, such as obstructive sleep apnoea (see Chapter 9), causing daytime sleepiness.

Determining how much sleep a person obtains is relatively straightforward—it is simply a matter of adding up the total number of hours slept in each 24-hour period. However, to prevent unnecessary concern, it is worth repeating that the average figure of 7–8 hours of sleep required for an adult is only a general guide. Some people need more than this ('long sleepers') while others function perfectly well on less—some on much less ('short sleepers'). It is important not to worry if you need less sleep than other people. It is only a problem if you are sleepy or affected in some other way during the day.

Poor-quality sleep can be more difficult to recognize. Repeatedly waking during the night (see Chapter 7 for possible reasons) will be obvious if you stay awake long enough to remember that you have done so. On the other hand, you will not know about brief moments of waking or fragmentation by brief arousals where you do not actually wake up. If it is necessary to examine this possibility, special sleep recordings (see Chapter 6) can be performed.

For general purposes, whether or not you are getting enough good-quality sleep can be judged mainly from the way that you feel during the day, starting from when you wake up in the morning.

## Signs of unsatisfactory sleep

Signs suggesting that your sleep is unsatisfactory and that it needs to be improved are listed in the box below. Some indicate excessive sleepiness, while others are features of insomnia or some other sleep disorder.

# Signs of unsatisfactory sleep

## Getting up in the morning

- Always having to be woken up (and possibly feeling irritable at being woken).

- Great difficulty waking up and getting ready for work or other activities.

- Feeling unrefreshed after a night's sleep.

## During the day

- Feeling drowsy, rubbing your eyes and yawning, eyes becoming unfocused, eyelids drooping, and head nodding.

- Actually falling asleep while doing something active (including driving or during conversation), indicating a more severe degree of sleepiness.

- Taking repeated naps during the day or feeling the need to do so.

- Repeatedly needing strong coffee or some other stimulant substance in an attempt to stay awake.

- Falling asleep in the evening, especially during activities that are not usually conducive to sleep.

- Falling asleep readily after only a small amount of alcohol.

- Feeling a strong need to sleep in late at weekends.

## At night

- Feeling desperate to get to bed early and then going to sleep almost as soon as your head touches the pillow.

- Conversely, persistently taking more than 30 minutes to get to sleep each night ('onset insomnia').

- Waking repeatedly during the night ('sleep maintenance insomnia').

- Waking early in the morning after very little sleep and not being able to go back to sleep ('early morning waking').

- If your bed partner tells you that you snore loudly, gasp, choke, or stop breathing while asleep.

**Other signs**

The following are problems that might be the result (at least partly) of insufficient or poor-quality sleep.

- Feeling constantly exhausted or fatigued with everything, even minor things.

- Loss of interest in activities that you previously found enjoyable.

- Becoming emotionally remote from family, friends, and colleagues.

- Not being able to concentrate, remember things, or think clearly.

- Making lots of mistakes at work or at home, or having lots of accidents.

- Feeling easily upset, depressed, vulnerable, or picked on.

- No longer feeling able to cope with things in general.

# Distinguishing between sleep disorders and other conditions

It is important to point out that disturbed sleep is by no means the only cause of the signs described in the box. These complaints can also result from:

- physical ailments, such as anaemia or an underactive thyroid gland;

- psychiatric disorders, such as depression or anxiety; or

- chronic fatigue syndrome (CFS)—also known as myalgic encephalomy-elitis or ME—which produces similar complaints, although some people diagnosed with CFS might actually have an undiagnosed sleep disorder that is the cause of their daytime symptoms.

A fundamentally medical or psychiatric condition should not be mistaken for a primary sleep disorder. Conversely, as discussed further in Chapter 12, some people whose symptoms are actually the result of a sleep disorder may wrongly be diagnosed as having depression, CFS, dementia, or some other condition.

As psychological problems (such as being stressed or depressed) can be either the cause of disturbed sleep or a consequence, it is necessary to decide which came first. Obviously, this will show whether help is needed mainly for the psychological problem or for the sleep disorder. Ideally, help should be provided for both at the same time. Improved sleep is likely to help you to cope with other difficulties.

# 6

# Sleep problems and their underlying causes (sleep disorders)

## ➜ Key points

- There are only three basic sleep problems; not sleeping well, sleeping too much, and behaving unusually or having strange experiences at night. However, there are many possible causes of these problems (i.e. sleep disorders).

- It is essential to identify the underlying sleep disorder because each requires its own form of treatment.

- Identifying the disorder involves careful questioning and sometimes special investigations.

## ✖ Myth versus fact

✖ **Myth**: If you don't sleep well, it's just one of those things and you have to put up with it.

❶ **Fact**: Nothing could be further from the truth. Careful enquiry will almost always reveal the reason why you are not sleeping well. This could be any of number of things. Once identified, the cause should be able to be treated effectively.

# Finding the cause of your sleep problem

Much of what has been said already shows that it is important to find out which of the various possible causes is responsible for someone not sleeping well. Such causes range from a minor illness or change of circumstances that will soon improve to serious conditions requiring intensive treatment.

As described in later chapters, there are many types of sleep treatments. Which one is most appropriate for a particular person depends on the underlying cause of their sleep problem. Unfortunately, the underlying cause might not be considered, even when professional advice has been sought. No one would say that difficulty breathing is an illness in its own right for which there is only one type of treatment, but something similar to this might happen in the case of difficulty sleeping, for example. That being so, sleeping tablets should rarely be prescribed for insomnia (see Chapter 8) or stimulant drugs for sleepiness (see Chapter 9) without regard to the many possible explanations and which of them applies in the individual case. The many forms of parasomnia (see Chapter 10) also call for different types of advice and treatment.

A person might have more than one sleep complaint, but there are only three basic sleep problems, which are:

- not sleeping well (insomnia);

- being too sleepy during the day (excessive sleepiness or hypersomnia); and

- behaving in unusual ways or having strange experiences at night (parasomnias).

However, a basic distinction needs to be made between a sleep problem (or complaint) and the cause of the problem, i.e. the underlying sleep disorder. Each of the three basic sleep problems can be the result of many possible causes.

The precise sleep disorder must be identified for each person (bearing in mind that more than one disorder might be present) because this determines the type of advice or treatment that should be chosen.

## Assessing someone with a sleep problem

To find out the cause of your sleep problem, your family doctor (and any one else you might need to see) will have to consider a number of points. It is obvious that this will take time—a few brief enquiries will not be adequate. Some of the main questions to be answered are as follows:

- What exactly do you feel is wrong with your sleep?

- What are your main worries about not sleeping well?

- When did the sleep problem begin and what has happened about it since?

- Has the problem been linked to you being ill or stressed in any way?

- Do you sleep better at weekends or on holiday?

- Is there anything else that helps you sleep better or seems to make you sleep worse?

- Is there anyone else in the family with a sleep problem and, if so, what type? Some sleep disorders run in families, for example, sleepwalking and other arousal disorders (see Chapter 10).

- In what ways has your sleep problem affected you and other people?

- Have you had any treatment to help you sleep better? What exactly did it involve? Did it work?

- Have you tried anything else yourself and did that help?

- Have you suffered from any illness or disorder recently (including depression or other psychological condition)?

- Have you recently taken any drug treatment for any ailment or other problem? Are you taking anything at the moment?

It will also be important to check on your sleep habits, your sleeping environment, habits that can disturb sleep, and your daily activities in general.

The following box provides a framework of items and questions to help you to review the main features of your typical sleep–wake pattern over each 24-hour period. It is useful to start with your evening meal and then work your way around the clock. You can compare this information with the signs that suggest unsatisfactory sleep (see Chapter 5).

# Your usual 24-hour sleep–wake pattern

## Evening

- What time is your last meal?

- What do you do between then and getting ready for bed? Is there a wind-down period as bedtime approaches?

- Do you fall asleep before bedtime?

- Do you have coffee late in the day?

- Is any sleep medicine taken?

- Do you use alcohol to get to sleep?

## Going to bed

- What is your bedtime routine?

- What time do you go to bed?

- What time do you go to sleep?

- What you do or experience before getting to sleep?

- Is the bedroom conducive to sleep?

- What you do if you can't get to sleep?

## During the night

- If you wake in the night, how often, for how long, and for what particular reason, if any?

- If your partner keeps you awake, in what way?

- What you do if you can't get back to sleep?

- Do you snore or have other breathing difficulties when asleep?

- Do you have strange experiences or behave in unusual ways during the night?

## Waking

◆ What time do you finally wake up?

◆ Do you have to be woken up? How?

◆ Do you find it very difficult to wake up? Are you irritable at being woken up? Do you feel a strong urge to get back to sleep?

◆ Do you feel that you have had enough sleep or not?

◆ Do you have unusual experiences before waking up properly?

◆ How much sleep will you have had before finally waking up?

## Daytime

◆ If you suffer from fatigue, drowsiness, or falling asleep, how often and for how long?

◆ Do you sleep in late at the weekend to catch up on sleep lost during the week?

◆ Do you have concentration difficulties or memory problems?

◆ Do you feel irritable or depressed?

◆ Have you lost interest in things?

◆ Do you have difficulties at work?

◆ Do you have problems at home?

◆ Do you have strange experiences during the day such as feeling weak?

# Other enquiries and tests

## What do other people have to say?

Although the person with the sleep problem is generally best placed to know the answers to most of these questions, other people (including your bed partner, other family members, and even friends) might have useful details to add.

◆ For some sleep disorders (such as those involving snoring, groaning, jerking movements during sleep, or sleepwalking), it is often your bed partner who brings the problem to light and persuades you to seek help.

◆ Family, friends, or workmates might be aware of how sleepy you are during the day or that your behaviour has changed.

◆ In the case of children (whose sleep problems may affect their parents' sleep; see Chapter 11), parents and the children themselves are the main source of information, although siblings, teachers, and possibly others may have made important observations.

## Keeping a sleep diary

Sometimes it is helpful to keep a sleep diary every day (see the following example) for, say, 1–2 weeks or possibly longer. Information collected in this way will overlap with that which you have collected retrospectively for each typical 24-hour period as described earlier. However, keeping a systematic record day by day can provide useful additional information, such as your general pattern of sleep and wakefulness, and various other factors that might consistently affect your sleep.

## Questionnaires

Sleep questionnaires for you (or, in the case of children, parents) to complete can be useful.

◆ Some ask questions about your sleep and its possible disorders in general.

◆ Others concentrate on particular aspects such as breathing problems in sleep or your degree of sleepiness (see Chapter 9).

◆ Yet other questionnaires are concerned with your beliefs and attitudes to sleep, which, if mistaken or unhelpful, might need to be corrected (see Sleep education in Chapter 8).

## Polysomnography

In some cases, hospital investigations may be necessary. One possibly useful investigation, depending on the sleep problem, is polysomnography (PSG), which consists of recording brain activity and other physical measures during overnight sleep and sometimes during the day. This is usually done in a hospital in a special sleep recording room.

### Example of a page from a sleep diary

| Day/date | |
| --- | --- |
| Time woke/woken. | |
| Time got up. | |
| How did you feel on waking? Did you feel rested as if you had had a good sleep? | |
| Did you feel tired or did you actually sleep at any time today? | |
| What did you do in the hour before bed? | |
| Time to bed. | |
| Time to sleep. | |
| Please describe any difficulties falling asleep, including why (if known) and what you did (if anything) to try to get to sleep. | |
| Time and length of periods awake during the night. | |
| Please describe anything else that happened during sleep/the night (for example, snoring or nightmares). | |
| Times of breakfast, lunch, and dinner. | |
| Anything else unusual, day or night. | |

PSG involves having small disc-like electrodes attached painlessly, usually with glue, to the scalp (an electroencephalogram), the side of the face (an electro-oculogram to record eye movements), and under the chin (an electromyogram to measure muscle activity). Other measurements might be needed depending on what sleep disorder is suspected. For example, breathing will need to be monitored carefully if obstructive sleep apnoea (see Chapter 9) is a likely possibility, or leg movements if it is thought that they are frequent and interfering with sleep (also see Chapter 9). In some cases, depending on the type of recording needed, PSG can be carried out at home using a miniature portable recording device.

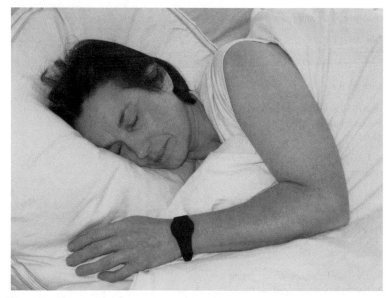

**Figure 6.1** Photograph of a person wearing an actometer

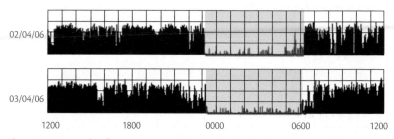

**Figure 6.2** Example of an actometry printout showing little movement during sleep

The degree and type of daytime sleepiness can be measured by means of a multiple sleep latency test. In this test, you are given the chance to fall asleep in the quiet surroundings of the sleep laboratory during PSG. This is repeated five times during the day. Sleepiness is measured as how long it takes you to fall asleep each time. People with narcolepsy for example (see Chapter 9) will go to sleep very quickly and will enter rapid eye movement (REM) sleep much sooner than is usual.

## Actometry

If all that is needed is the overall pattern and timing of sleep and being awake, this can be provided by means of actometer (or actigraph) recordings. This entails wearing a wrist-watch type of device (at home or elsewhere) that measures body movements by day and night (see Figures 6.1 and 6.2).

## Audio-visual recordings

Overnight recordings of this type can be useful for establishing the nature of unusual behaviour related to sleep (see parasomnias, Chapter 10) and for assessing the degree of breathing difficulty during sleep, especially in obstructive sleep apnoea (see Chapter 9).

Usually these recordings need to be performed in a special room in hospital, but sometimes useful information can be obtained by means of audio-visual recording systems alone that can be operated at home, including the use of domestic recording equipment.

## Other tests and assessments

Depending on what might be the cause of your sleep problem, blood tests of one sort or another may be appropriate, or other assessments of a physical or psychological nature in an attempt to decide the most appropriate advice or treatment in your case.

# 7

# Not sleeping well (insomnia)

## ➔ Key points

◆ Insomnia is the most common sleep problem, affecting 30% or more of adults.

◆ Insomnia can be transient (lasting several days), short term (lasting a few weeks), or chronic (lasting months or years).

◆ The many potential causes of these forms of insomnia tend to be different, each cause requiring its own type of advice or treatment.

◆ Treatment with sleeping tablets is rarely appropriate.

## Definition of insomnia

Most people who complain of insomnia have the following difficulties, quite possibly in combination.

◆ They have difficulty falling asleep.

◆ They are not able to go back to sleep easily if they wake in the night.

◆ They wake early in the morning without being able to go back to sleep at all.

◆ They are not refreshed by their sleep, no matter how long they have slept.

Everyone has the occasional night of sleeping badly without the need for help or advice. However, surveys have repeatedly shown that about 30% of young and middle-aged adults are affected often enough by insomnia for it to be a significant problem. This figure is much higher (at least 50%) in elderly people and also in some other groups who are at special risk of disturbed sleep (see Chapter 11).

People who show a lifelong ability to function perfectly well on relatively little sleep ('short sleepers') are not considered to suffer from insomnia.

It is worth repeating that the problem of insomnia cannot be considered a condition or diagnosis in itself. It is a symptom and its cause needs to be discovered in each individual.

There are many possible causes of insomnia, which, for the most part, are different, depending on how long the problem has lasted (see box below). There may be more than one cause, particularly in elderly people.

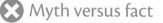 **Myth versus fact**

❌ **Myth**: Everyone has difficulty sleeping sooner or later. You just have to put up with it.

❗ **Fact**: It is true that most people probably have occasional brief spells of not sleeping well, perhaps for no obvious reason. However, if the problem persists, there is likely to be an identifiable cause that should be dealt with because of the potentially serious consequences of persistently not sleeping well.

❌ **Myth**: Some people haven't slept for years.

❗ **Fact**: This cannot be true, else they would not have survived! People who say this think they haven't slept because they only remember the times when they have woken in the night and have forgotten the rest of the time that they have, in fact, been asleep.

## Misperceptions about insomnia

Before considering the causes of insomnia, it should be mentioned that a proportion of people with this complaint are actually sleeping normally. This may well be the case with some elderly people but also others who, for example, habitually worry about themselves. This over-concern about their sleep can be the result of:

◆ having unrealistic expectations of how much sleep they need;

◆ only being aware of the times when they wake up in the night (as mentioned above, occasional waking is normal in everyone—a problem only arises if it is not possible to get back to sleep again); or

◆ feeling the need for sympathy or attention—as a personality trait or because of upsetting circumstances.

Obviously, it is essential that a distinction is made between 'genuine' insomnia and that which is more imagined. This might require the type of special sleep recordings described in Chapter 6. If it is confirmed that a person's sleep is indeed normal, it is essential that the right kind of advice or other help is provided for what—to that person—has been a real problem.

## Main examples of the causes of insomnia according to how long the problem has lasted

Note that there may be more than one cause at any one time.

### Transient insomnia (lasting from days to a week or two)

◆ Worry about a coming challenging experience.

◆ Upset about a family matter or work-related issue.

◆ Excitement about going on holiday.

◆ Sleeping somewhere new.

◆ A brief illness.

◆ Jet lag.

### Short-term insomnia (lasting a few weeks)

◆ A longer illness.

◆ More persistent worry about problems at work or at home, or about being ill.

◆ A longer-standing upset involving personal relationships.

◆ Bereavement.

### Chronic (long-term) insomnia (lasting months to years)

◆ Unresolved causes of short-term insomnia.

◆ Poor sleep hygiene.

- ◆ Having come to associate bed with being awake rather than with being tired and ready for sleep ('conditioned' or 'learned' insomnia).

- ◆ Mistiming of your sleep including delay of your sleep phase or going to bed too early, causing early-morning waking.

- ◆ Medical or psychiatric conditions (or their treatment) that disturb sleep.

- ◆ Restless legs syndrome.

- ◆ 'Childhood insomnia'.

# Types of insomnia

Insomnia can be classified as 'transient' (lasting several days to perhaps a week or two), 'short term' (lasting up to several weeks), and 'chronic or long term' (lasting months or even years).

## Transient insomnia

Most people experience this at some time or other. Common causes include worrying about a coming interview, a family dispute or some other stressful or upsetting experience, perhaps at work, or a short-lived illness. Alternatively, you might find it difficult to sleep because you are excited (for example, about going on holiday) or because you have to sleep somewhere new or in a noisy or otherwise unsatisfactory place. Jet lag also causes transient insomnia.

As these causes are mostly temporary, sleep can be expected to return to normal before long without the need to do anything special about it.

As in other types of sleep disturbance, good sleep hygiene is important in minimizing the effects of influences that disturb sleep (see Chapter 8). It is best first to see if improving your sleep hygiene will solve your sleep problem. This is better than taking sleeping tablets.

If it is highly likely that you will have serious trouble sleeping for several nights because the circumstances causing the disturbance cannot be altered, taking a short-acting sleeping tablet (prescribed by your doctor) for, at most, several nights might be justified (see Chapter 8). Not only can this help to prevent daytime problems, but it might also avoid a brief sleep problem developing into a long-term difficulty.

## Short-term insomnia

Sleeping badly might persist for several weeks if some of the factors that cause transient insomnia are more severe or long-lasting. Examples include a longer drawn-out illness, persistent worries about being ill, problems at home, or difficulties at work.

Being upset about personal relationships can have the same effect and so can bereavement; the latter can affect your general well-being for a long time if the grieving process is impeded.

The kind of help and advice that you need will depend on your particular circumstances, but it is important that you are helped to understand the cause of your particular problem. Again, you might be helped during difficult times by the short-term use of sleeping tablets. Advice on how to reduce your stress can also be helpful. Once more, good sleep hygiene is important.

## Chronic (long-term) insomnia

It has been estimated that 10% or more of adults suffer from insomnia that has lasted months or even years. The longer the sleep problem has persisted, the harder it may be to see how it started, partly because the picture can become confused by the psychological effects of not sleeping well.

For example, your attention might become focused on feeling tired, exhausted, or miserable during the day, rather than on the sleep problem that is responsible. Possibly, the original cause no longer exists, but bad sleep habits have become established, maintaining the difficulty.

Sometimes there is a definite cause but one that is not easily identified (and which will continue to be overlooked) unless you are asked very specific questions by your doctor. In particular, if you are elderly, you may have more than one cause of your sleep problem.

# Causes of chronic insomnia

## Unresolved causes of short-term insomnia

Probably the most common reason for persistently not sleeping well is some form of enduring psychological difficulty or concern not severe enough to amount to a psychiatric illness. Some people are more liable than others to feel particularly stressed about the everyday problems of living. Things prey on their mind when they go to bed and try to sleep, or when they wake during the night. If unresolved, worries that can cause transient or short-term insomnia can have more prolonged effects.

Lying in bed worrying or thinking about the day's events at work or at home, or about health and other issues, makes it difficult to relax enough to sleep. A vicious spiral is often set up. Realizing that it is difficult to get to sleep, and worrying about the effect that this will have the next day, raises your level of anxiety still further and makes the problem worse.

As just described, some people have a mistaken idea of how much sleep they need or misinterpret how much sleep they are actually getting. Such ideas can be an unnecessary source of concern, which itself then causes a sleep problem. Your quality of sleep can suffer as a result, causing the daytime problems described in Chapter 2.

## Poor sleep hygiene

Sleep hygiene does not refer to personal cleanliness at night! Poor sleep hygiene occurs when your circumstances and habits prevent you from sleeping well. Examples include a sleeping environment that is not conducive to sleep, napping too much during the day, and an excessive intake of caffeine.

The principles of sleep hygiene (see Chapter 8) are an important part of overall advice for anyone with a sleep problem, whatever its cause or nature. Sometimes, all you need to do to sleep better is to improve your sleep hygiene.

## Conditioned or learned insomnia

This refers to the habit of having come to associate being in bed with being awake and feeling distressed, rather than being content, relaxed, and ready for sleep. You may then become preoccupied by your sleep problem. This can develop, whatever the original cause of not sleeping well. If you sleep better in a new environment that is not associated with sleeping badly, this suggests that you have conditioned insomnia.

## Mistiming of sleep

Sleeping at the wrong time can result in difficulty getting to sleep and other problems during the day, including excessive sleepiness (see Chapter 9). There are various possible reasons why you may sleep at the wrong time. Some are due to circumstances beyond our control, such as jet lag or having to work shifts; others are a consequence of our chosen lifestyle.

Jet lag should be a problem only for a matter of days, whereas shift work can produce long-standing difficulties. Both of these conditions are covered in the section dealing with groups of people who are especially prone to sleep disturbances (see Chapter 11).

Going to sleep very early is likely to lead to waking early in the morning and finding it impossible to go back to sleep because your need for sleep has been met. There is a tendency for this to occur in elderly people, because of a change in either their body clock or their lifestyle ('advanced sleep-phase syndrome' or ASPS; see also Chapter 11). Gradually delaying bedtime can help to correct ASPS. Otherwise, exposure to bright light for at least half an hour in the evening can help to re-time the period of sleep (again, perhaps with the help of a light box in severe or resistant cases). Melatonin has also been used. See Chapter 11 for other possible causes of sleep problems in the elderly.

The sleep of people who abuse alcohol or drugs can become so disorganized that it is split into short periods throughout the day and night, sometimes with no two days alike. This is likely to cause additional psychological problems. The following additional cause of sleep mistiming deserves further mention because it appears to be quite common.

## Delayed sleep-phase syndrome (DSPS)

This condition can develop when you persistently work late or socialize until the early hours and therefore get into the habit of not going to sleep until late. You may then find that you cannot go to sleep earlier, no matter how much you want to. This is because the body clock controlling your sleep and wakefulness has become reset.

Although common in adolescents, this situation can arise at any age, including in young children who have habitually not gone to sleep until very late for whatever reason. Some people with DSPS share a family tendency for the sleep phase to be delayed, although this is relatively rare. The extent of the delay can be considerable—you might not go to sleep until the middle of the night or later. Once asleep, your sleep is then sound, but it will not have lasted for long enough for you to feel refreshed by the time you have to get up for work or your other usual daytime activities.

This lack of sleep makes it very difficult to wake up (even with the aid of an alarm clock) and you feel tired and exhausted, especially during the first part of the day, after which the tiredness may wear off. You may well feel that you have to sleep for part of the day. When the opportunity arises, especially at weekends, you are likely to sleep in very late, but this simply perpetuates the abnormal sleep–wake pattern during the week. DSPS can occur at any age, but is thought to be particularly common in adolescents (see Chapter 11).

## Treatment of DSPS

This problem can be difficult to put right, but it is important to do so because its effects can be serious. The main things that should not be done are as follows:

- Try not to 'catch up' on your sleep by sleeping in late at weekends (this perpetuates the abnormal sleep pattern by confusing your body clock).

- Do not simply go to bed much earlier—this associates being in bed with being awake.

- Do not use alcohol to get to sleep, or stimulants to be alert during the day.

Instead, there are various ways of resetting the body clock to a more appropriate time; this is known as 'chronotherapy'.

- If the sleep-phase delay has been relatively modest, bedtime can gradually be brought forward.

- In severe cases, where it is impossible to get to sleep until many hours later than you want to, it may be necessary to move the sleep phase all round the clock (by, say, 3 hours at a time each 24 hours) until the ideal sleep time is reached. This needs much organization and commitment by all involved, and for it to work you need to be motivated to make the lifestyle changes required.

Other measures that can also be helpful are as follows:

- Expose yourself to bright light after waking up (possibly with the aid of a 'light box', which simulates sunlight) to suppress the output of melatonin around that time.

- Ensure that the bedroom is in darkness as bedtime approaches (to encourage melatonin output).

- Take synthetic melatonin (see Chapter 8) at night-time to further promote the onset of sleep.

- Strict sleep hygiene, including consistent times for going to bed and getting up, is important.

Some young people (and, for that matter, some others) may be found to be motivated to maintain their abnormal sleep phase and persistently sleep in late, for example to avoid unwelcome daytime experiences or commitments at school or at work.

### Other circadian sleep–wake cycle disorders

Gross disturbances of sleep–wake patterns can occur with abuse of alcohol and other substances, causing profound psychological effects that might not be seen as the result of disrupted sleep.

Sleep–wake cycle disorders caused by lack of light perception (see Chapter 3), and their unwelcome effects, are a problem in blind people.

## Medical conditions and treatments

Brief illnesses can easily disturb sleep while they last, as part of feeling generally unwell or as a result of being uncomfortable or distressed. Sleep usually returns to normal once you have recovered.

Medical conditions that last a long time are likely to disturb sleep for an equally long period, unless something can be done to prevent this happening. It is important to try to do so, because loss of sleep makes it much more difficult to cope with other problems.

◆ Prostate enlargement or diabetes can cause repeated trips to the toilet at night.

◆ Other medical conditions, such as eczema or certain types of arthritis, can cause discomfort or pain at night.

◆ Heart conditions, breathing disorders (for example, obstructive sleep apnoea, asthma, or emphysema), and ulcers or other gastrointestinal disorders also often disturb sleep in one way or another—including by worrying about being ill.

◆ Certain medications can disturb sleep. Examples include some treatments for high blood pressure, heart complaints, breathing disorders, or depression. You should tell your doctor if you notice any change in your sleep when you start taking a particular medication or when the dose is increased.

The important point here is that, as far as possible, the doctor who is looking after you should try to help you to sleep better. For example, this may be achieved by adjusting the treatment you are receiving for your medical condition. In addition (or if no improvement in your basic condition is possible), your doctor should offer specific treatment for your sleep disturbance.

## Restless legs syndrome

This is another not-uncommon cause of chronic insomnia. In the evening or when lying down to sleep at bedtime (and sometimes on waking during the night), some people experience creeping, crawling, prickly, or otherwise uncomfortable feelings in their legs, which they attempt to relieve by moving them, for example, by walking about the bedroom or rubbing them vigorously.

This is called 'restless legs syndrome' (RLS). It can cause serious difficulty getting to sleep and much distress. It may also explain some cases of 'growing pains' in children. RLS often runs in families. Sometimes it occurs during pregnancy or in people with a physical condition such as iron-deficiency anaemia or rheumatoid arthritis. Some medications can also cause the problem or make it worse.

Usually, RLS is accompanied by abnormal leg movements during sleep, called 'periodic limb movements in sleep' (PLMS), a possible cause of poor-quality sleep and daytime sleepiness (see Chapter 9), although it can also occur separately. Various drug treatments are available for both of these conditions.

## Psychiatric disorders

In addition to the many medical conditions linked to disturbed sleep, there are also a number of psychiatric problems that affect sleep, i.e. psychological illnesses requiring psychiatric treatment, as distinct from common reactions to the problems of everyday living discussed earlier. Again, the sleep complaint is often difficulty getting off to sleep or not sleeping soundly, although some people find that they are excessively sleepy or have other sleeping difficulties.

There are many ways in which psychiatric conditions are frequently complicated further by sleep disturbance:

◆ Being anxious or depressed is likely to make it difficult to fall asleep and frequently sleep is also disrupted.

◆ Anxious people can have panic attacks during the night (see Chapter 10).

◆ Depressed people often wake early in the morning and cannot get back to sleep.

◆ As well as sleepiness, insomnia can be one of the features of seasonal affective disorder or SAD (see Chapter 9).

◆ Insomnia and other sleep disorders (especially nightmares) commonly develop after severe trauma as part of post-traumatic stress disorder (PTSD; see Chapter 10).

◆ Insomnia and other forms of sleep disturbance frequently complicate misuse of alcohol or other substances, including withdrawal effects when you stop taking them.

In many of these circumstances, night-time can become associated with anxiety, depressive thoughts and dread, or frightening experiences to the extent that it becomes even more difficult to sleep. If the underlying condition is successfully treated, the person will probably begin sleeping better. In the case of depression, however, it should be noted that certain antidepressant drugs can have a stimulating effect and worsen insomnia. Clearly, careful choice of treatment by your doctor is essential.

## Childhood-onset insomnia

There are some people who seem to have suffered from insomnia since they were young children ('childhood-onset insomnia'), presumably because of a constitutional difficulty with sleeping. This rather ill-defined condition should not be assumed to be the cause of an adult's sleeping difficulty. It is important that other possible explanations are explored.

## Primary insomnia

You may come across the term 'primary insomnia' in various books and articles. This is not another kind of insomnia. It is a term used to refer to difficulty sleeping that is not the result of a medical or psychiatric condition or of the various disorders caused by mistiming of the sleep period. It usually refers to 'idiopathic' or 'childhood-onset insomnia' (that is, insomnia of constitutional origin, rather than caused by another disorder).

## Multiple causes of insomnia

There may well be more than a single reason for not sleeping well. For example, a man might be unhappy with his job, finding it frustrating or too stressful. In addition, it may not pay enough to meet his family commitments, especially if a new baby arrives or his wife is no longer able to be a second wage earner for some other reason. He may resort to drinking too much as an escape, which, together with being somewhat overweight, could cause him to develop some degree of obstructive sleep apnoea (see Chapter 9). His snoring disturbs his wife's sleep and causes further tensions in an already fraught marital situation. This then contributes further to his disturbed sleep, which increasingly causes him to feel worse during the day and to perform less effectively at work.

In such complex circumstances, it is necessary to try to disentangle these various factors and see how one feeds into another. Inevitably, treatment and advice will be complicated but essential for the good of all concerned.

# 8

# Treatments for insomnia

## → Key points

- The choice of treatment for insomnia should be based on the cause of the problem, i.e. the underlying sleep disorder.

- Principles of good sleep hygiene are important for helping anyone to sleep well, but they are also valuable in combination with more specific treatments, depending on the cause of your insomnia.

- Sleeping tablets have a very limited part to play in the treatment of insomnia and can be harmful. They are no substitute for treating the underlying cause of not sleeping well.

- Coming off sleeping tablets can be troublesome and needs careful supervision.

- Sleeping aids bought over the counter are of doubtful value and can cause daytime problems.

- With professional supervision, psychological and behavioural treatments can be very effective.

## The importance of finding the cause of your insomnia

As already stressed, it is essential that the basic cause of insomnia is identified and treated, whenever possible. However, you probably do not need to see your doctor if your sleep problem has lasted for only a short time and is a normal understandable reaction to your circumstances—such as those mentioned earlier as causes of transient insomnia.

Jet lag is one of the few exceptions to this rule where prescribed
the form of a short course of sleeping tablets (or possibly mel:
justified (see Chapter 11).

## Sleep hygiene

This term refers to basic ways of helping you to sleep well. The principle
good sleep hygiene apply to anyone, but they are particularly useful for tho.
with a sleep disorder, usually in addition to the appropriate specific treatment.
Observing these principles is the best way to help yourself and can be enough
to resolve a sleep problem.

Advice about sleep hygiene is set out in the box below. Each point will not
apply equally to everyone. It is important to consider what applies to you.

---

### Advice on sleep hygiene

#### Ways to help you sleep better

- Sleep in a comfortable bed.

- Make sure that the bedroom is dark, quiet, and the correct temperature.

- Only use your bed for sleep and sexual activity.

- Have regular times when you go to bed and when you get up.

- Go to bed only when you are tired.

- Take regular exercise every day, eat a healthy diet, and keep fit.

- Try to experience sunlight outdoors, preferably at the same time each day.

- Some people are helped to go to sleep by having a warm bath or a milky drink before bedtime, reading or listening to quiet music in bed, visualizing a pleasant scene, or concentrating on a relaxing or monotonous experience.

- Be sure to arrange help for your sleeping partner if he keeps you awake, for example, by snoring, jerking, or constantly moving about.

---

## Things to be avoided

- Caffeine-containing drinks (see Chapter 7) late in the day because of their stimulating effect.

- Smoking, especially near bedtime (nicotine is also a stimulant).

- Large meals late at night.

- Stimulating activities (including exercise) just before going to bed.

- Using your bedroom as a place of entertainment or work.

- Taking your problems to bed or trying to make plans in bed. It is best to set aside a time in the early evening for such things.

- Trying to force yourself to sleep.

- Becoming preoccupied by difficulty getting to sleep.

- Having a clock nearby to keep looking at to see how long you have been unable to get to sleep.

- Lying awake in bed for more than half an hour (see Chapter 7).

- Inappropriate napping during the day (see Chapter 3).

- Using alcohol to help you sleep.

- Using your own or someone else's sleeping tablets.

## ❌ Myth versus fact

❌ **Myth**: An alcoholic drink at bedtime is a good way of helping you to sleep well.

❗ **Fact**: It may help you to get to sleep but is likely to disturb your sleep later in the night.

❌ **Myth**: If I can't get to sleep, I should stay in bed and try harder.

> ❗ **Fact:** This is likely to make matters worse because you will probably become tense and frustrated. Being in bed will become associated with being awake instead of going to sleep.
>
> ❌ **Myth:** If you sleep longer at weekends, you can make up for loss of sleep during the week.
>
> ❗ **Fact:** It doesn't work that way. Regular bedtimes and waking up times are important, otherwise your circadian body clock gets confused.

It is important to be realistic about your need for sleep. Not everyone needs 8 hours of sleep, and having the occasional poor night's sleep is normal.

Being in bed must be associated in your mind with being relaxed and ready for sleep rather than lying there awake and stressed, as this can easily become a habit. These points are discussed further later in this chapter in the section on psychological treatments.

## Medication

### General points about hypnotic drugs

Various drugs have been used to try to help people sleep better. They all have the effect of dampening certain brain systems, or activating others, that are involved in the process of sleeping. Although drugs are still often prescribed for insomnia, their use is not often justified, especially in elderly people. They should be used only as a last resort in particularly distressing circumstances. They are no substitute for dealing with the basic reason for not sleeping well, such as depression or the other possible explanations mentioned in the previous chapter.

> ❌ ## Myth versus fact
>
> ❌ **Myth:** The only treatment for insomnia is sleeping pills.
>
> ❗ **Fact:** This is far from the case. In fact, the use of sleeping pills is rarely appropriate. Instead, depending on the reason why you are not sleeping well, one of a wide range of treatments other than medication can be used.

In addition, taking sleeping tablets can give rise to serious problems. The effects can last into the next day ('hangover effects'), making you feel tired, muddle-headed, or confused, and impairing your ability to concentrate, remember things properly, and make decisions or perform skilled actions such as driving or operating machinery.

Sometimes they cause unwelcome changes in personality such as irritability, over-excitement, and lack of drive.

As your body gets used to the drug after perhaps only a few weeks, increasing doses are often needed to produce the same effect on sleep ('tolerance'). Many people develop the habit of taking sleeping tablets long term, which is difficult to break ('psychological dependence').

## Withdrawal effects

People taking the commonest sleeping pills—benzodiazepines (see later)—also often become physically dependent and experience severe difficulties if they try to come off them because their body has become used to having the drug in their system. This can happen within a few hours of stopping a short-acting benzodiazepine, but can take much longer than this with a longer-acting type. These 'withdrawal effects' consist of distressing physical and psychological symptoms including anxiety, depression, confusion, loss of appetite and body weight, tremors, sweating, ringing in the ears, and possibly abnormal perceptions. In addition, insomnia and disturbing dreams may well develop. It is easy to confuse these effects on sleep with the original sleep complaint and to conclude that you need to keep taking the tablets when this is not the case.

Abrupt withdrawal of benzodiazepines can induce particularly serious effects including psychotic states and convulsions. There are a number of other possible risks and complications. Hypnotic drugs can depress breathing and should be avoided by people with respiratory disorders including obstructive sleep apnoea (see Chapter 9). Also, they can worsen the effects of alcohol and other drugs that depress brain activity, including some of the over-the-counter products sold as sleeping aids.

## Substance misuse

Misuse of benzodiazepine drugs in particular is common in people who abuse alcohol or other substances. Very serious effects include death from overdose and (in those who inject) gangrene and infection with hepatitis and human immunodeficiency virus (HIV).

## Safe use of hypnotic drugs

In the very few circumstances where the use of sleeping tablets is justified, the risks of hangover effects, tolerance, and dependence can be reduced if the drug is:

- one with an action lasting for a short or medium length of time (less than 8 hours);

- taken in the lowest effective dose for the shortest possible time (for example, for two or three nights in the case of a sudden traumatic event, or for up to 2–3 weeks at most in longer periods of distress); or

- used intermittently (such as one night in three).

## Elderly people

In general, older people, for example over the age of 65, are particularly vulnerable to the side effects and some of the other complications of hypnotic drugs. They eliminate the drugs more slowly, their breathing can be depressed by benzodiazepines more readily, and they may take other medications (and possibly a night-time alcoholic beverage) with which sleeping tablets can interact.

Therefore, the elderly should take no more than half of the usual adult dose of any sleeping tablet that is thought absolutely necessary. Too high a dose can cause over-sedation with confusion, wandering at night, unsteadiness and the risk of falls (possibly causing fractures), and other accidents at home, outside, or when driving. Difficulty concentrating or remembering things caused by the medication can be mistaken for dementia.

## Stopping sleeping tablets

As described above, you should be prescribed sleeping tablets only for very good reasons in exceptional circumstances. Routine repeat prescriptions are rarely, if ever, justified. For those who have been on sleeping tablets for a long time, it is generally best to withdraw them. This needs to be done gradually under the careful supervision of your doctor with psychological support. There is evidence that this approach can often be successful and that people then function better without their sleep deteriorating.

# Types of hypnotic drugs

The box below lists various drugs (and their classification) that have been used in the treatment of insomnia.

# Medications used for insomnia

Trade (or proprietary) names (where used) are shown in brackets.

## Benzodiazepines

Short acting (effects lasts a few hours):

- Loprazolam.

- Lormetazepam.

Medium acting:

- Lorazepam (Ativan).

- Temazepam.

Long acting:

- Nitrazepam (Mogadon).

- Diazepam (Valium).

## Z drugs

- Zopiclone (Zimovane).

- Zolpidem (Stilnoct).

- Zaleplon (Sonata).

## Other drugs (see text for limited or doubtful usefulness)

- Sedative antidepressants.

- Barbiturates.

- Chloral hydrate.

- Chlormethiazole.

- Melatonin.

- Antihistamines.

- Herbal preparations.

Both benzodiazepines and Z drugs (so-called because each of the members of this group begins with the letter 'z') act on receptors to increase the inhibition of certain pathways in the brain.

## Benzodiazepines and Z drugs

The harmful effects and complications discussed above have been reported more often in people who have taken benzodiazepines rather than Z drugs, which disturb sleep physiology to a lesser degree. However, Z drugs are not free of risks.

Of the individual benzodiazepines, sudden withdrawal of the short-acting variety is particularly liable to cause 'rebound insomnia' as part of their withdrawal effects. Hangover effects are more likely with a long-acting benzodiazepine.

Zolpidem and zopiclone have similar effects to the benzodiazepines with regard to the onset of sleep and its duration. However, because it is so short acting, zaleplon will only help you get to sleep at bedtime, although it has also been used sometimes to help someone to return to sleep if they wake in the night.

## Other drugs for insomnia

If your insomnia is caused by depression, you may be prescribed an antidepressant drug that also has a sedating effect (for example, amitriptyline, mirtazapine, or trazodone) and which, therefore, should help you to sleep if taken at night.

Antidepressant medication can be helpful if there is good reason to believe that someone's sleep problem has been caused by depression. However, there is no direct evidence that antidepressants help you sleep better if this is not the case.

The relationship between depression and disturbed sleep is a two-way process. Depression can cause sleep problems but, conversely, disturbed sleep can cause depression. It is important to try to establish which way round applies in any particular case. The sequence of events should indicate whether the emphasis in treatment is best placed on the depression or the sleep disorder, although it may be appropriate to combine both approaches to some degree.

Barbiturates, chloral hydrate, and chlormethiazole are older drugs that are generally best avoided because of harmful side effects.

## 📄 Case study

### Insomnia

Megan, a 40-year-old woman, saw her GP because, although she found it difficult to get to sleep and had kept waking in the night for several years, her sleep problems had become much worse in the last few months. She also complained of increasing difficulty over the same period in coping with the demands of her part-time job as a shop assistant.

From talking to Megan and her husband (who was also seen in order to obtain possible additional information) and examining her, the GP felt that there was nothing to suggest that there was any physical reason (including breathing difficulties at night) why she was not sleeping well, and there was no obvious evidence of poor sleep hygiene.

However, it came to light that, for some time, Megan had been feeling depressed and lacking in energy and enjoyment of her home life. She had lost interest in her hobbies and her job, as well as her friends. Also, her appetite had become poor and she had lost 10 pounds in weight.

She did not connect her present problems with the fact that she had suffered previous bouts of depression after the birth of her second child and some years before that for no apparent reason. On both of these occasions, she had been prescribed antidepressants, which had seemed to help. Both her mother and her sister had experienced similar problems.

Megan was treated initially with a low dose of a sedating antidepressant, which improved her sleep somewhat. Within 2 weeks of an increase in the dose, she began to sleep much better and to feel much improved generally in herself, gradually regaining her enthusiasm for her home life, work, and leisure activities.

## Melatonin

Melatonin is a hormone mainly produced naturally in the pineal gland within the brain. It has widespread effects on the body, including helping to control the circadian sleep–wake rhythm (see Chapter 3).

Synthetic melatonin has been used to treat sleep disorders where there is mistiming of the sleep period, such as in jet lag or shift work, and possibly other sleep–wake cycle disorders including those in blind people (see Chapter 3). Its usefulness in other sleep disorders is debatable, although, in keeping with its short duration of action, it does seem to be helpful sometimes, including in some children who have difficult getting off to sleep.

There is little information about the long-term side effects of melatonin or about appropriate dosage. Also, as there have been some concerns about the content and purity of commercially available melatonin, it is important that, as far as possible, only a quality-controlled form should be used.

You are advised not to drive or perform other tasks requiring concentration for 4–5 hours after taking melatonin because it might make you sleepy and less alert. Only the lowest effective dose should be used.

Melatonin is not licensed for use in the UK, but can be prescribed by doctors for individuals whom they think might benefit. It is not available in shops in this country and has usually been obtained 'over-the-counter' abroad, by mail order, or via the internet.

### Other treatments

The use of exposure to sunlight or the use of light boxes ('phototherapy') to correct the mistiming of the sleep phase (and thereby the insomnia associated with, for example, delayed sleep-phase syndrome; see Chapter 7) has already been mentioned. Other conditions involving insomnia that can successfully be treated with phototherapy include shift work (see Chapter 11) and some forms of depression.

## Treating yourself

This is not a good idea! Self-medication with non-prescribed substances or products is not advisable because this stands in the way of discovering the cause of your sleep problem.

Consumption of alcohol is not an appropriate way of helping you to sleep. Using alcohol may help you get off to sleep but the effect does not last and, once the sedating effect of the alcohol has worn off, your sleep is likely to be disturbed, perhaps with vivid dreams caused by a rebound of increased rapid eye movement (REM) sleep later in the night ('rebound insomnia'). Also, you may have to get up more to go to the toilet.

Over-the-counter products to help you sleep often contain sedative antihistamines (such as promethazine and diphenhydramine), but it is not obvious that they are effective; they may well cause hangover effects and you can experience rebound insomnia when you stop taking them.

Other products contain herbal preparations such as valerian. Again, the value of these substances is uncertain and there is some risk of unwelcome effects.

## Psychological treatments for insomnia (including cognitive–behavioural therapy)

### General points

◆ Various psychological treatment programmes are available for people who have suffered insomnia for some time. Psychological and behavioural factors are often responsible for insomnia becoming long lasting and the programmes are designed to help you overcome these influences. The term 'cognitive–behavioural therapy' reflects the psychological and behavioural factors underlying the sleeping problem.

◆ The term 'psychological treatments' here should not be confused with psychiatric treatment, which is concerned with mental illness of one sort or another. General counselling alone is not an adequately specific sleep treatment, although it may have a part to play in overall help for someone's personal problems.

◆ Psychological treatments for insomnia, without the use of medication, can be helpful but they are not used as much as they should be because they are not known about and used sufficiently by healthcare professionals. Your doctor should be able to advise where this type of help is available.

◆ A programme of psychological treatment needs to be designed specially for each individual. Some aspects involve self-help measures, but the programme as a whole will usually require the help of a psychologist or someone else with special knowledge of the psychological approaches to insomnia.

◆ As with other treatments, you need to persist with this form of treatment to give it a proper chance to work. You might need support and encouragement from a therapist or adviser to do this, especially as your sleep problem could become worse before it gets better.

◆ General sleep hygiene (see earlier this chapter) is important in providing a background of self-help measures for use in combination with the specific psychological treatment procedures, some of which are based on individual sleep hygiene principles.

The following are the main forms of psychological treatment that have been used for insomnia, either individually or in combination. There is some overlap in the basis of some of these approaches. Advice on such procedures and other behavioural treatments is best obtained from a professional with experience of using them.

## Sleep education

Many people have mistaken beliefs about or unhelpful attitudes towards their sleep, which can be a cause of not sleeping well or can make their pre-existing sleep problem worse. For example, you might believe that you should be able to fall asleep immediately on going to bed or that everyone needs 8 hours of sleep at night.

Being given basic information about sleep, including changes with age and also individual differences in sleep requirements, can be helpful and even therapeutic, especially if such information corrects misunderstandings that have given rise to anxieties about your own sleep or that of family members. Knowing that there are effective treatments for sleep disorders is also likely to be reassuring.

## Cognitive therapy

Cognition is the process of thinking and understanding. Combined with sleep education, cognitive therapy aims to correct mistaken ideas and negative thoughts about sleep that can make insomnia worse.

Some people worry that they are helpless to control their ability to sleep (perhaps because of the ageing process) and, therefore, that they will inevitably be adversely affected during the day, perhaps indefinitely. Similarly, you may be convinced that all your daytime problems are caused by not sleeping as well as you would like and that the situation is hopeless. These unhelpful thoughts can be changed by acquiring more accurate information about sleep, but, in particular, by replacing them with more positive or accurate attitudes and beliefs.

## Stimulus control

This treatment aims to reduce your anxiety about sleep by making sure that you associate your bed and bedroom with sleep so that they are re-established as a stimulus (or cue) to go to sleep. Ways in which this might be done have already been touched on in the list of sleep hygiene principles, but, where insomnia has already become a serious problem, it might be necessary to work on these aspects of treatment more thoroughly. The main ways of doing this are by paying particular attention to the following:

- Go to bed only when you are sleepy.

- Use your bed only for sleep and sex. Do not use your bedroom as a place for TV entertainment, for example, or work-related activities.

- Do not fall asleep elsewhere in the house.

If you have not fallen asleep after 20 minutes or so, get up, go to another room, and do something that is not stimulating, and go back to bed only when you do feel sleepy (you might need to do this more than once in a night). The other sleep hygiene principles, including regular bedtime and waking-up times as well as avoiding daytime naps, are also important.

## Sleep restriction

This treatment aims to increase your 'sleep efficiency'—the ratio of the time you spend asleep to the time you are in bed. It works by restricting the time that you spend in bed to the time when you are actually sleeping rather than lying there awake.

If, for example, you lie in bed for 8 hours but spend the first 2 hours awake, you would start the treatment by not going to bed until 6 hours before the time you have to get up. This can be difficult because you need to be firm with yourself about staying up late and initially you usually get even less sleep than before because you might not get off to sleep quickly at first.

However, it is important to stick to the new routine, to carry on getting up at the usual time and not to nap during the day. Soon it should be possible to fall asleep more quickly and to sleep soundly. The time you spend in bed can then gradually be lengthened until you are getting a satisfactory amount of sleep at night.

## Relaxation

This treatment aims to teach you how to relax when you want to. It can help you overcome the tension and feelings of anxiety that are common in people who sleep badly. The various methods include muscle relaxation exercises at bedtime, breathing exercises, and other ways of preventing your mind from being too active.

## Other psychological methods

These include:

◆ ways of teaching you how to block out unwelcome thoughts that are inter-fering with sleep ('thought stopping'); and

◆ 'paradoxical intention' in which, by trying to stay awake, you actually increase the likelihood that you will fall asleep by diverting your thoughts away from the fear that you will not be able to do so.

📄 Case study

### Cognitive–behavioural treatment for insomnia

Anna, a 36-year-old woman with two teenage boys, had suffered for several years from an inability to get to sleep at night. She had begun to sleep badly for the first time when her father died and, although she even-tually got over her bereavement, her sleep pattern had never returned to normal. Various over-the-counter sleeping aids had not helped and some had made her feel more tired during the day. She became increasingly upset at feeling generally unwell, anxious, and unable to cope properly at home.

Anna's GP could find no physical reason for her poor sleep and, being reluctant to prescribe sleeping tablets, referred her to a sleep disorders clinic. There it was felt that Anna did not have a depressive illness or any other primary psychiatric disorder, and that her low spirits and anxiety were the result of inadequate sleep caused by not being able to get to sleep until about 2 a.m. and then having to get up about 6 a.m. to rouse the children and help them get ready for school. There was no evidence of any other sleep disorder.

In the first session with the psychologist who was part of the team at the sleep clinic, it soon became clear that Anna had certain unhelpful beliefs about her sleep. She had become convinced that she had lost control over her ability to sleep, would be unable to sleep well again, and that, as a result, she would never be able to look after her family properly. Also, as she lay in bed unable to go to sleep, she had constant thoughts that her lack of sleep would eventually harm her physical health and, therefore, that her insomnia was damaging her entire life.

Subsequent sessions were concerned with teaching Anna ways of combating these negative thoughts, which she was able to manage with practise. In addition, a programme combining stimulus control and sleep restriction measures was set up. The main overall aim was to remove the link in Anna's mind between lying awake in bed for long periods and feeling agitated and distressed about not being able to sleep, and to substitute it with the association of being in bed and feeling relaxed enough to sleep.

Anna was encouraged to go to bed only when she was sleepy (even though initially this meant waiting until the early hours of the morning) and then to get up at the required time during the week and at the equivalent time at weekends, and not to take naps during the day.

Although she found this very difficult initially, with her husband's help she persisted, and within a fortnight she was able gradually to move her bedtime earlier and still get to sleep readily. This allowed her to obtain enough sleep to feel much better during the day. This improvement has been maintained for the past 2 years.

# 9

# Excessive sleepiness

## ➡ Key points

◆ Excessive sleepiness—enough to cause serious difficulties—is common but is often not viewed as a medical problem for which help is available.

◆ There are many causes, each requiring a specific type of treatment.

◆ The main causes are not getting enough sleep, not sleeping soundly for various reasons, and conditions in which a person sleeps to an abnormal degree.

◆ Obstructive sleep apnoea is a common cause of poor-quality sleep and excessive sleepiness at all ages, but there are many other possible explanations to consider.

◆ In addition to being psychologically and socially disabling, excessive sleepiness can be hazardous, for example by causing accidents.

## ✖ Myth versus fact

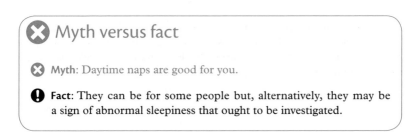

✖ **Myth**: Daytime naps are good for you.

❗ **Fact**: They can be for some people but, alternatively, they may be a sign of abnormal sleepiness that ought to be investigated.

# Identifying excessive sleepiness

Everyone is likely to have times when they feel tired for no obvious reason. However, if asked, a surprising number of people will say that they are regularly far too sleepy, often to the extent that it affects them seriously.

Excessive sleepiness can take the form of:

◆ feeling tired and sleepy, and lacking in energy;

◆ actually falling asleep repeatedly during the day; and

◆ feeling the need to sleep for excessively long periods overnight with great difficulty getting up in the morning.

These forms can occur in combination. Excessive sleepiness can have a number of unwelcome effects on your life. Everyday activities can become a burden, enjoying yourself becomes a thing of the past, your emotional life is upset, and your performance during the day may be impaired, possibly causing accidents at work or while driving.

Despite these serious consequences, relatively few people who are excessively sleepy seek medical help. Their condition may well be mistaken by themselves or by other people for laziness or boredom. On the other hand, it may be thought that they are suffering from a primarily psychological or medical disorder, or even from failing intellect if the effects are severe.

Conditions where the main problem is excessive sleepiness tend to be different from those in which lethargy or fatigue is the most prominent feature (without necessarily needing to sleep excessively), such as chronic fatigue syndrome or CFS (also known as myalgic encephalomyelitis or ME), depression, or a medical illness of one sort or another. However, the distinction may not always be clear; if there is any doubt, it is best to consult your doctor.

Again, it is worth remembering that some people need more sleep than others without necessarily having anything wrong with them. However, if you are persistently not at your best during the day or have shown other signs of a sleep disorder (see Chapter 5), you should obtain professional advice.

## How sleepy are you?

> ### ✖ Myth versus fact
>
> ✖ **Myth**: Some people are just sleepy heads. There's not much to be done about it.
>
> ❗ **Fact**: If you are persistently very sleepy, something should (and usually can) be done to correct it, because the consequences can be serious.

The Epworth Sleepiness Scale (see box below) is a simple but useful way of judging how sleepy you are. A score of 8 or less can be considered normal, 9–16 is mild-to-moderate sleepiness, and over 16 indicates that you are severely sleepy. If you score over 8, professional advice is required.

To get a thorough assessment of your sleepiness and its cause, you might need to undertake the kind of special sleep studies described in Chapter 6. These can be provided by the sleep disorders clinics that now exist in the UK and elsewhere. You can be referred to one of these by your doctor (see Chapter 13).

> ### The Epworth Sleepiness Scale
>
> How likely are you to doze off or fall asleep in the following situations, in contrast to just feeling tired? This usually refers to your way of life in recent times. Even if you have not done some of these things recently, try to work out how they would have affected you. Use the scale to choose the most appropriate number for each situation:
>
> 0 = would never doze
>
> 1 = slight chance of dozing
>
> 2 = moderate chance of dozing
>
> 3 = high chance of dozing

| Situation | Chance of dozing |
|---|---|
| 1. Sitting and reading. | _____ |
| 2. Watching television. | _____ |
| 3. Sitting inactive in a public place (for example, the cinema or a meeting). | _____ |
| 4. As a passenger in a car for an hour without a break. | _____ |
| 5. Lying down to rest in the afternoon (when circumstances permit). | _____ |
| 6. Sitting and talking to someone. | _____ |
| 7. Sitting quietly after lunch without alcohol. | _____ |
| 8. In a car, while stopped for a few minutes in traffic. | _____ |
| **Total score** | _____ |

## Causes of excessive sleepiness

The influences that determine how sleepy you feel (your 'sleep drive') were mentioned in Chapter 3. There are many possible reasons why you might be excessively sleepy (see box below). Some are more common than others, and some more obvious than others. Finding the explanation in each individual case is best left to family doctors or specialists familiar with the characteristic signs of each of the possible causes. Treatment varies widely depending on the cause.

## Possible causes of excessive daytime sleepiness

### Insufficient sleep

◆ Accumulated 'sleep debt'.

◆ Mistiming of sleep.

## Poor-quality sleep

- Stress and worry.

- Medical or psychiatric conditions (and some treatments).

- Obstructive sleep apnoea and other breathing disorders.

- Periodic limb movements in sleep.

- Some work-related conditions.

## An abnormal need for sleep

- Narcolepsy.

- Idiopathic hypersomnia.

- Some forms of depression (including seasonal affective disorder or SAD)

- Kleine–Levin syndrome.

- Menstruation-related sleep disorder.

- Other medical conditions.

- Drug abuse.

### Insufficient sleep and sleep debt

The most obvious cause of persistent sleepiness is lack of sleep. Therefore, it is important to know whether your hours of sleep at night are so reduced (by persistently going to bed late, not being able to get off to sleep, being awake during the night, or waking early in the morning) that you are likely to be sleepy or otherwise affected during the day.

The longer you suffer from loss of sleep, the more you build up a 'sleep debt' (see Chapter 2) and the worse you will be during the day. As already empha- sized, it is important to identify the reasons why your sleep is reduced in these ways so that the correct solution can be found. The various conditions in which there is mistiming of your sleep cause both insomnia and excessive daytime sleepiness. Delayed sleep-phase syndrome, which is common in adolescents but can occur at other ages (see Chapter 7), is a prominent example of this.

## Poor-quality sleep

You may be excessively sleepy because, even though you are getting the right number of hours of sleep, the quality of your sleep is poor due to repeated interruptions (see Chapter 5). If your sleep is constantly interrupted, the normal pattern of overnight sleep (discussed in Chapter 3), with a balance between non-rapid eye movement (NREM) and rapid eye movement (REM) sleep, is lost and NREM sleep fails to reach its deep, restorative levels. The quality of your sleep can suffer for the following reasons.

### Stress and worry

If you are stressed and worried about everyday matters, your sleep is likely to be restless and broken. However, as discussed in the last chapter, it is important to distinguish between stress (or depression for that matter) as a *cause* of poor sleep and as a *consequence* of poor sleep. Clearly, the help required is different in these two situations. In the second situation, emphasis should be placed on treatment of the sleep problem in the expectation that the feelings of being stressed will be reduced when sleep improves.

### Medical and psychiatric conditions and treatments

The various causes of insomnia (in addition to stress and worry) discussed in Chapter 7 may wake you repeatedly during the night or disturb your sleep without you actually waking up. This fragmentation of sleep can also be caused by some of the treatments used in medicine and psychiatry. Some psychiatric drug treatments, such as tranquillizers, may well cause daytime sleepiness directly.

### Obstructive sleep apnoea (OSA)

> ## ❌ Myth versus fact
>
> ❌ **Myth**: Snoring is a joke or at worst a nuisance.
>
> ❗ **Fact**: It's not funny if someone else's snoring keeps you awake. More to the point, it can be a sign of a serious condition (obstructive sleep apnoea) that needs to be treated.

OSA is a medical cause of excessive sleepiness that deserves special mention. It is a common condition affecting people of all ages (including children) and can cause serious problems. About 4% of adult men, rather less than that in women, and possibly 2% of children suffer from OSA. Women are particularly susceptible after the menopause. All groups are at increasing risk as obesity becomes more common. Unfortunately, only a small minority of people with this condition seek advice from their doctor, perhaps because few realize that OSA is the reason why they feel tired or exhausted during the day, or why they have other problems.

In OSA, the back of the throat (which may already be compressed by fat deposits in the neck) blocks off (obstructs) repeatedly during sleep. This happens because the throat muscles relax. Consequently, the walls of the throat are repeatedly sucked in and the airway is narrowed. This blocking off causes breathing to stop, perhaps for many seconds, because air cannot pass into the lungs.

Each interruption of breathing ('apnoea' from the Greek for not breathing) limits the supply of oxygen to the brain and, at the same time, the level of carbon dioxide in the blood rises. The overall disturbance of your breathing causes your brain to almost wake you up, or to actually do so although usually without you being aware that it is happening. Breathing then starts up again with a large intake of breath that rattles the soft palate and nearby structures, producing a loud snore. The person might also make gasping or choking sounds, moan, mumble, or move about, sometimes violently. Some people wake up at the end of an apnoeic episode feeling frightened or confused, perhaps with the sense that they are suffocating.

In adults, OSA is associated with being overweight and having a thick neck. However, there are other causes such as conditions in which the upper airway is congenitally narrowed, as in Down syndrome or in other conditions in which the structure of the face and back of the throat is not normal. In contrast, the usual explanation in children is enlarged tonsils and adenoids, although obesity is increasingly also becoming a cause.

## Effects of OSA

Episodes of apnoea can happen hundreds of times a night, interrupting sleep each time, so that sound, refreshing sleep is impossible. As a result, people can be badly affected during the day. They may have great difficulty waking up and may have a headache when they do.

During the day, they are likely to be very sleepy and unable to concentrate, remember things, or make decisions properly. They may also feel irritable, constantly exhausted, anxious, or depressed. In severe cases, they may be thought to be suffering from dementia. Performance at work is likely to decline and the person may even lose their job. Relationships with family can suffer, interest in sex can be lost, and some men become impotent. Overall, the quality of life can be seriously impaired.

OSA is also a dangerous condition. Sufferers have been shown to have more driving accidents than other people as a result of falling asleep at the wheel. They also have more accidents at work because of the difficulty they have paying proper attention to what they are doing. OSA can cause high blood pressure and other serious health problems including heart failure, heart attacks, and strokes. Obviously, there are many reasons why OSA should be recognized and treated at as early a stage as possible.

### Snoring

Snoring still tends to be regarded as something of a joke or (more seriously) a nuisance to other people whose own sleep is affected by it.

Snoring does not necessarily mean that you have OSA. Many people snore to some extent without it being of serious significance other than being troublesome to the sleeping partner or others nearby. However, if you snore loudly and persistently, especially if your breathing is repeatedly interrupted, as described above, and if you are sleepy or affected during the day in the other ways mentioned, then OSA is highly likely.

If your partner, or a member of your family, seems to have these symptoms, they may well be unaware of it unless told. It is important to encourage them to seek the advice of their doctor who will be able to refer them to a clinic specializing in OSA.

### Investigating OSA

Investigations for OSA include careful assessment of the sleep problem and general condition, as well as studies in which sleep and breathing overnight (including blood levels of oxygen and carbon dioxide) are carefully monitored. The degree of sleepiness during the day (and other daytime problems) also needs to be assessed. There are various sleep centres in the UK where these assessments can be carried out, most of which are in local hospital departments of respiratory medicine.

### Treating OSA

Most people with OSA can be treated and the results can be dramatic, possibly transforming their lives. So-called continuous positive airway pressure (CPAP) is the main form of treatment for adults with OSA. This involves wearing a mask over the nose and mouth at night, through which air is blown under pressure to keep the throat open, preventing it from repeatedly collapsing.

Other important aspects of treatment include the following:

◆  Weight reduction should be undertaken in the high proportion of OSA sufferers who are overweight.

- Avoid alcohol near bedtime, as it can depress breathing and make apnoeas worse.

- Do not using sleeping tablets as these can have the same effect as alcohol.

- Avoid smoking, as nicotine can narrow the upper airway.

- Any other medications that can impair breathing during sleep, such as sedative drugs, should be used with care.

- People who suffer from OSA only when they are lying on their back can be helped by being encouraged to sleep on their side (for example, by placing pillows behind their back).

- Sometimes physical abnormalities that interfere with breathing can be removed surgically—such as nasal polyps or (in children) enlarged tonsils and adenoids.

- Good sleep hygiene, including avoiding loss of sleep, in general is also important (see Chapter 8).

Various other measures are sometimes used, including mechanical devices (such as appliances that hold your jaw forward during sleep or that dilate the nasal passages) and antidepressant-type medications that reduce REM sleep, as OSA occurs only or mainly in this type of sleep.

## 📄 Case study

### Obstructive sleep apnoea

For a year, James, aged 38, had suffered from headaches, mainly in the morning, that were especially bad after waking up. Various headache pills had not been helpful and he began to worry that he might have something seriously wrong with him such as a brain tumour. He went to his GP, whom he had not seen for some years, to ask whether he should be seen by a hospital specialist.

The GP was concerned that the patient was very overweight and that his blood pressure was high. When asked, James admitted to being very tired during the day and said that he often struggled to stay awake at work. His wife said that he was much more irritable and forgetful than he used to be and that he snored so loudly that she often went to another room to try to sleep. She also described his breathing as being very irregular at night.

An appointment was made at the local hospital department of respiratory medicine. There, the patient's score on the Epworth Sleepiness Scale was found to be 19, indicating a severe degree of daytime sleepiness. Overnight polysomnography in hospital with audio-visual monitoring demonstrated a severe degree of OSA, with many interruptions of his breathing, which were associated with a lowering of his oxygen blood level. Each interruption ended with a loud snore.

Treatment with CPAP was started, together with advice about weight reduction, the avoidance of alcohol near bedtime, and other sleep hygiene principles. Soon, his breathing during the night improved including (to his wife's relief) no further snoring. In addition, his headaches cleared up and he became much more energetic and less forgetful during the day. His blood pressure also improved. By means of a diet and taking more exercise, he lost 3 stone in weight. He has now maintained these improvements for the past 2 years.

### Other conditions that can affect breathing during sleep

In addition to OSA, there are other conditions, in both adults and children, in which breathing is affected during sleep, impairing its quality and leading to tiredness and other problems during the day. Frequent asthma attacks at night can do this and also, for example, muscular dystrophy and previous poliomyelitis, which can cause weakness of the breathing muscles.

### Periodic limb movements in sleep (PLMS)

Some people's limbs (generally their legs) tend to jerk repeatedly during the night ('periodic limb movements') and this can disrupt their sleep without them waking up. If this happens a lot during the night, the quality of your sleep may be poor and you will not be refreshed, causing you to be sleepy during the day.

It is the bed partner who may be only too well aware of these movements as a cause of their own sleep disturbance.

PLMS can exist in its own right or as a feature of other sleep disorders such as OSA. It can also accompany various neurological conditions including some encountered in children. PLMS can co-exist with restless legs syndrome (see Chapter 7). Various drug treatments have been used for both of these conditions.

## Work-related conditions

Night-shift workers have special difficulties with sleep that arise from a combination of insufficient and poor-quality sleep when they are off duty. This is covered in more detail in Chapter 11.

People in other occupations whose work pattern means that their sleep is consistently affected in these ways are likely to be sleepy during the day as a result. For instance, junior doctors can be sleepy as a result of long hours of duty and irregular sleep patterns. Other people prone to disrupted and poor-quality sleep include those who care for chronically ill relatives (including those with disturbed sleep–wake rhythms caused by dementia) and parents of sleepless young children (see Chapter 11).

# An abnormal need for sleep

Some sleep disorders cause you to spend much more time asleep than is normal.

## Narcolepsy
### General features

This neurological condition, which occurs in both adults and children, is caused by a defect in the hypocretin (or orexin) system, which is involved in controlling the transmission of impulses in some parts of the brain. Affected people are unable to resist falling asleep repeatedly during the day for relatively short periods ('sleep attacks'). They also have poor-quality sleep at night, and so feel generally sleepy.

They may also experience sudden episodes of muscle weakness (without feeling faint or blacking out), which are usually triggered by a strong emotional experience such as laughter, anger, or fear—this is called 'cataplexy'. Cataplexy can cause them to collapse to the ground if they become weak all over, or the episodes may be less obvious—for example, only their jaw may drop or their head fall forward. Sometimes, they simply feel weak or unsteady.

In some people with narcolepsy, there are also temporary episodes of 'sleep paralysis' in which they cannot talk or move as they are falling asleep or when they are waking up. They might also have vivid and sometimes frightening dream-like experiences when dozing or falling asleep ('hypnagogic hallucinations' from the Greek for 'sleep' and 'leading to') or when waking up ('hypnopompic hallucinations' from the words for 'sleep' and 'sending away').

Cataplexy, sleep paralysis, and hypnagogic and hypnopompic hallucinations happen when aspects of REM sleep (paralysis and dreaming; see Chapter 3) occur while you are still awake. The combination of these features and the abnormal sleepiness is called the 'narcolepsy syndrome'.

It is important to know that sleep paralysis or such hallucinations also occur in many people who do not have narcolepsy or any other serious condition (see Chapter 10).

### Diagnosis

Narcolepsy quite often begins in childhood or adolescence, although it is frequently not recognized for several years after it first begins. It can usually be diagnosed from the presence of the various symptoms just described, plus overnight sleep recordings and a multiple sleep latency test (see Chapter 6). A special test (human leucocyte antigen or HLA test) can also be helpful and, where there is doubt about the diagnosis, an estimation of the level of hypocretin in the cerebrospinal fluid (which is low in narcolepsy) may be justified.

### Treatment

Narcolepsy tends to be a life-long condition, although carefully chosen and supervised treatment can be helpful in reducing the symptoms. This consists of medication that makes you feel more alert (for example, modafinil or amphetamines) to combat the excessive sleepiness, and other drugs (such as some that are also used for depression) to treat the cataplexy, sleep paralysis, and hallucinations, if necessary. Sometimes other drugs are used. In the future, it may be possible to correct the low levels of hypocretin in the brain by taking this substance as medication.

Planned naps once or twice a day (preferably including a mid-afternoon nap), stimulating activities, and the avoidance of obesity can be helpful, as well as attention to general sleep hygiene principles.

Incidentally, a recent development is the use of modafinil in healthy people to try to increase their powers of concentration or to reduce their need for sleep. It has yet to be seen to what extent this is feasible or, indeed, desirable.

All concerned (parents, other children, teachers, and workmates) should have the condition explained to them to prevent misunderstandings. Career advice is also important because it may not be possible to treat the condition fully and it is likely to persist.

# 📄 Case study

## Narcolepsy

A 14-year-old girl called Rachel had been well until the last 3 months when she had begun to feel very sleepy most of the time, actually falling asleep repeatedly during the day, even when she was active such as when talking or eating a meal. She also had attacks of suddenly feeling weak and falling to the ground without losing consciousness, or her mouth would sag open so that she could not speak for a few seconds.

In addition, Rachel reported that, when drifting off to sleep at night, she felt that objects in the room changed shape or the dimensions of the room seemed to be altered. Sometimes these experiences were accompanied by being unable to move her body for up to 20–30 seconds. Understandably, she had become afraid to go to bed at night.

Rachel was referred by her GP to the local neurologist who could find no abnormality when he examined her physically. He remarked that she seemed to be an accomplished girl in many ways, without any psychological problems other than being concerned about her condition. Her score on the Epworth Sleepiness Scale was 17, which indicated a high degree of sleepiness.

Sleep studies in hospital were arranged. The results showed that she fell asleep very rapidly and almost immediately into REM sleep. This, and the results of her HLA test, confirmed the GP's strong impression that she was suffering from narcolepsy syndrome.

Treatment with medication, and advice about taking planned daytime naps, as well as sleep hygiene, were soon largely effective. It was explained that Rachel would probably need to continue treatment indefinitely. The nature of her condition was explained fully to her parents, friends, and teachers.

Excessive sleepiness can be an intrinsic part of certain other disorders (described below), some of which seem to be basically the result of a person's constitution. These conditions do not have the characteristic features of narcolepsy.

## Idiopathic hypersomnia

People with this condition have great difficulty waking up properly in the morning, despite sleeping soundly at night and, in most cases, for a prolonged period. They can remain drowsy, confused, and unsteady for some hours—a condition known as 'sleep drunkenness'—and may take long unrefreshing naps during the day.

Idiopathic hypersomnia, which usually begins in early adult life at the latest, can run in families. Stimulant drugs, such as modafinil, can be helpful for this troublesome and often persistent condition.

## Depression

Although most depressed people suffer from insomnia, quite a number complain that they are excessively sleepy in a way that may not be wholly the result of a lack of sleep. Antidepressant medication usually leads to improved sleep as the depression lifts.

Seasonal affective disorder (or SAD), which develops in winter, is characterized by depression, fatigue, and overeating, as well as excessive sleepiness or other sleep disturbances (see also Chapter 7). Treatment includes exposure to bright light using a 'light box', which simulates the intensity of sunlight that is needed for this form of treatment to be effective.

## Kleine–Levin syndrome

People with this uncommon disorder, which usually begins in adolescence, go through periods (lasting days, weeks, or longer) during which they are asleep most of the day and night, before sleeping and behaving normally again, perhaps for several weeks. This cycle continues to repeat itself.

When, during a sleepy period, the patient is briefly awake, behaviour is often abnormal and out of character, such as overeating or being disinhibited in various ways (perhaps sexually).

It is important for it to be explained to all involved that this is a medical illness and not a psychological disorder. Medication has little part to play but, fortunately, the condition tends to improve eventually.

## Menstruation-related hypersomnia

Some women become very sleepy as a result of their menstrual cycle (see Chapter 11).

## Other medical conditions

Excessive sleepiness can occur in a variety of neurological conditions in addition to those already mentioned, including:

◆ Parkinson's disease;

◆ head injury;

◆ some brain infections or tumours; and

◆ certain genetic disorders in which brain mechanisms involved in sleep and wakefulness are disturbed.

Other medical disorders having the same effect include underactivity of the thyroid gland and following glandular fever.

## Drug abuse

Various states of drug intoxication, as well as withdrawal from stimulant drugs, can cause excessive sleepiness.

# 10

# Disturbed behaviour and strange experiences at night (parasomnias)

## ➡ Key points

◆ There are many different ways in which behaviour and experience can be disturbed in relation to sleep.

◆ Many of these conditions mainly occur in children (who usually grow out of them), but others persist into or start in adult life.

◆ It is unusual for parasomnias to be caused by serious medical or psychiatric problems.

◆ Parasomnias can occur when going off to sleep or when waking up, in light non-rapid eye movement (NREM) sleep, in deep NREM sleep early in the night, or in rapid eye movement (REM) sleep usually later in the night. Some occur at various times of the night.

◆ It is important to know precisely the type of parasomnia because treatment (if needed) varies significantly from one type to another.

## ✖ Myth versus fact

✖ **Myth**: Nightmares and night (sleep) terrors are basically the same thing.

❶ **Fact**: Not so. They are different in a number of ways, including their causes and the type of advice and treatment required.

> ❌ **Myth**: You should wake up a sleepwalker.
>
> ❗ **Fact**: No. It is difficult to wake a sleepwalker and, if you manage it, he is likely to be confused and frightened.
>
> ❌ **Myth**: Eating cheese gives you nightmares.
>
> ❗ **Fact**: Research has shown that there is no support for this idea.

## Sleep is not always peaceful

Sleep is not always a relaxed, uneventful state. Often, various changes in behaviour or experiences take place during or in the period closely related to sleep. Sometimes these events are worrying to the person experiencing the parasomnia. On the other hand, he may not know what is happening because he is asleep at the time. So-called 'arousal disorders' (see later this chapter) are of this type.

The changes in behaviour or experience in the parasomnias can be very subtle, but others are dramatic and alarming to the individual or to anyone who witnesses them. However, especially in childhood, even dramatic events of this type do not usually mean that they are caused by something serious.

The box below lists various parasomnias in relation to the phase of sleep with which they are usually linked and, therefore, the time of night when they usually occur (see also Figure 3.1). It is essential that the episodes are correctly diagnosed and not confused with each other because the causes and treatments are very different. Distinguishing one type of parasomnia from another requires attention to detail. Sometimes, special sleep studies are needed (see Chapter 6).

## Some parasomnias in relation to the time of night when they usually occur

### When going to sleep

- Sleep starts.

- Hypnagogic hallucinations.

- Sleep paralysis.

- Rhythmic movements (for example, headbanging).

- Restless legs (sometimes also during the night after waking up).

## Early in the night (or later) in light NREM sleep

- Teeth grinding.

- Periodic limb movements.

## Early in the night in deep NREM sleep

- Sleepwalking.

- Sleep terrors.

- Confusional arousals.

## Later in the night in REM sleep

- Nightmares.

- REM sleep behaviour disorder.

- Sleep-related groaning.

## When waking up

- Hypnopompic hallucinations.

- Sleep paralysis.

## At various times of night

- Sleep talking.

- Bedwetting.

- Some medical parasomnias (e.g. certain types of epilepsy).

- Some psychiatric parasomnias (e.g. panic attacks).

# Parasomnias when going to sleep

## Sleep starts

Most people experience an occasional jerk of the body as they are dropping off to sleep ('hypnic jerks'), often associated with a feeling of tripping up or falling. Others hear what seems like a loud bang or explosion in their head (the 'exploding head syndrome'!) or see a flash of light. These jerks and sensory experiences are called 'sleep starts'. Although alarming, they do not mean that there is anything medically wrong.

## Hallucinations

Many children and some adults have 'hypnagogic hallucinations' in which they experience apparent changes in the size, shape, or colour of objects in the bedroom, or other odd and sometimes frightening perceptual changes when falling asleep. If they occur on waking up, these experiences are called 'hypnopompic hallucinations'.

## Rhythmic movements

A significant proportion of young children, often from infancy onwards, bang their heads rhythmically into the pillow or against their cot side at night ('headbanging'); others move rhythmically in some other way such as rolling from side to side. Sometimes they make noises in time with the movements.

Usually this happens when they are going to sleep or going back to sleep after waking during the night. One view is that these movements help in getting to sleep at bedtime or after waking during the night. Although they can seem strange, such behaviours (called 'rhythmic movements') usually occur in healthy children, and are not harmful and do not usually require treatment other than preventing injury from impact on a hard surface, for example by padding the cot sides. However, if they are a source of distress, embarrassment, or upset to other family members, the child can be given treatment.

Both medication and various psychological approaches have been used successfully, depending on the exact nature of the problem. Even with no treatment, rhythmic movements of this type almost always stop spontaneously by the age of about 3. Occasionally rhythmic movements at night occur in adults.

Similar rhythmic movements that occur during the day (rather than being related to sleep) are different from those just described in that they are often associated with severe neurological disorders.

## Sleep paralysis

A surprising number of people experience 'sleep paralysis' (sometimes accompanied by hallucinations) in which it is not possible to move or speak for several seconds up to a minute or so. This may be associated with a frightening feeling of not being able to breath even though, in fact, the muscles controlling breathing (and eye movements) are not affected. Each episode may stop of its own accord or by being touched, moved, or spoken to.

If hallucinations and sleep paralysis are not part of the narcolepsy syndrome (see Chapter 9), which is usually the case, these strange experiences in a drowsy state are almost always entirely normal and you can be reassured that there is nothing physically or psychologically wrong. However, if they are particularly worrying, they can usually be treated successfully with medication of an antidepressant type (without the person actually having a depressive disorder).

## Restless legs syndrome

This is another parasomnia that can occur in the period before falling asleep (see Chapter 7).

# Parasomnias early in the night (or later) in light NREM sleep

## Teethgrinding

Some people grind their teeth ('bruxism'), usually while they are sleeping lightly and mainly early in the night. However, it can also happen during later periods of light NREM sleep (see Figure 3.1). The grinding can be forceful enough to produce a loud noise (perhaps enough to disturb others trying to sleep nearby) and cause a headache or pain in the face. In severe cases, when the teeth are likely to be damaged, fitting a protective dental device can be helpful. If the teeth grinding is caused by stress, relaxation exercises, for example, may also help.

## Periodic limb movements in sleep

These involuntary movements (see Chapter 9) can occur in this stage of overnight sleep.

# Parasomnias early in the night in deep NREM sleep

## General features of arousal disorders (sleepwalking, sleep terrors, and confusional arousals)

These three types of arousal disorder episodes have many features in common.

- They usually happen early in the night (within about 2 hours of going to sleep) when deep NREM sleep or slow-wave sleep (SWS) from which these episodes arise occurs.

- Arousal disorders are, in fact, 'partial arousals' from deep sleep without actually waking up. The result is a combination of features suggestive of being both awake and asleep at the same time.

- These types of parasomnia often run in families for genetic reasons. Close blood relatives may have had one or other of these types of arousal disorder.

- In those who are predisposed this way, individual episodes may be triggered by factors such as loss of sleep, fever or other illness, stress, some medications, certain other sleep disorders such as obstructive sleep apnoea (OSA), and possibly alcohol.

- Arousal disorders occur mainly in children.

- Episodes stop after a few years in the majority of people but sometimes persist into adult life. Rarely, they begin in adolescence.

- They are usually infrequent and, for the most part, happen only once in any one night.

- Some children begin to have confusional arousals when they are very young, followed later by sleepwalking episodes, and then, in later childhood, they develop sleep terrors. Some arousal disorder episodes contain elements of more than one of these types.

- At times, an arousal disorder episode consists of elements of more than one type.

- Unusually, it seems, arousal disorders occur in combination with REM sleep behaviour disorder (see later this chapter). This is called 'parasomnia overlap disorder'.

## Sleepwalking

Sleepwalkers (sometimes called 'somnambulists') behave in a generally confused way, wandering around the house and doing inappropriate things like urinating into the wardrobe as if mistaking it for the bathroom. Some carry out quite complicated activities, even though they are still asleep. Provided the actions are familiar or habitual, they might, for example, make drinks or meals, wander outside the house, perhaps for long distances, or even drive a car.

Some people develop an eating disorder with excessive weight gain as a result of the amount of food that they consume while they remain asleep.

Although some sleepwalking episodes involve fairly controlled walking about ('calm sleepwalking') with eyes open and in a semi-purposeful (although often accident-prone) way, other people behave in a frenetic fashion ('agitated sleepwalking'), rushing about and crying out as if trying to escape from danger.

Sometimes sleepwalkers perform aggressive or destructive acts, causing injury to themselves or others, and sexual offences can be committed in the course of a sleepwalking episode.

A person may not know that anything has happened during an arousal disorder episode unless he wakes up at the end of it (as sometimes happens) or is told afterwards what he has done.

### Legal aspects

If antisocial acts are committed while genuinely asleep, the sleepwalker cannot be held legally responsible because, being asleep at the time, he did not know what he was doing. Similar considerations may apply in REM sleep behaviour disorder (see later this chapter).

On the other hand, a sleepwalker may be considered somewhat to blame if he puts himself at risk of having a sleepwalking episode by (from past experience) knowingly behaving in ways that are likely to trigger an episode such as missing a lot of sleep or consuming alcohol.

Guidelines have been suggested to aid the recognition of genuine sleepwalking in legal cases where this explanation for an illegal act has been used as a defence.

## Sleep terrors

In sleep terrors (sometimes called night terrors or 'pavor nocturnus'), behaviour is generally much more disturbed than in sleepwalking. Although appearing to be terrified (crying out or screaming, wide-eyed, pale, sweating, and seemingly trying to escape from danger), the person remains asleep and is not consciously distressed. After a short time, he will suddenly calm down and begin to sleep restfully again.

## Confusional arousals

Confusional arousals, seen mainly in very young children, are somewhat like sleep terrors in that the child appears to be confused and distressed while actually still asleep. Parents may be particularly alarmed to witness their child's apparent distress and need to be reassured that the child is not, in fact, suffering.

## Advice and treatment of arousal disorders

No attempt should be made to wake someone having an arousal disorder episode, despite the understandable urge felt (especially by parents) to comfort them. It is difficult to wake the person and, if achieved, it is then likely to frighten them. Instead, the episode should be allowed to run its (usually brief) course.

In cases where the sleepwalking takes an agitated form, or in the course of a sleep terror, there is a serious risk of accidental injury, for example from crashing through a bedroom window or falling downstairs. Therefore, it may be necessary to take precautions to make the environment safe in various ways such as keeping the bedroom door shut or fitting heavy curtains to the bedroom windows to prevent them breaking if the sleepwalker tries to escape by that route.

It is comforting to parents to know that their child is likely to grow out of his tendency towards these arousal disorders. In the meantime, the following suggestions about prevention and treatment are likely to help for both children and adults.

- It is important to avoid the triggering factors mentioned earlier, including aspects of good sleep hygiene.

- Practising good sleep hygiene is important.

- If psychological factors are thought to play a prominent part, treatment for emotional problems or ways of reducing stress may be helpful.

- If the child is not aware of his episodes at the time they occur, it may well be best not to tell him the details of them (especially if dramatic) to save him being worried about himself.

◆ If the child knows in general terms that he walks in his sleep, he should be reassured that other children have his kind of sleep problem and that he will almost certainly grow out of it.

◆ If sleepwalking or sleep terror episodes are frequent and occur consistently at about the same time of night, it may be possible to prevent them by waking the person shortly before one is due, keeping him awake for a few minutes, and then letting him sleep again. However, this form of treatment ('anticipatory awakening') needs to be carefully supervised, preferably by someone experienced in its use.

◆ Medication, such as a benzodiazepine (see Chapter 8), can also be used to a limited extent for severe cases or, for example, to avoid a child being embarrassed by having episodes when briefly away from home. This also needs careful supervision, preferably with the advice of a sleep specialist.

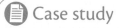 Case study

**Sleep terrors**

The parents of Sam, a 9-year-old boy, were worried about him going on a school trip away from home because, two to three times a week for the last few months, he had screamed out in the night and was found sitting up in bed looking extremely fearful.

This always happened about 90 minutes after Sam had gone to sleep. Each episode lasted for a few minutes (during which time they were unable to get through to him) before he settled down again. Sam had no recollection the next morning that anything had happened.

There seemed to be a tendency for these episodes to be more frequent if he was worried about something or if he was unwell with a cold or some other minor ailment. Sam was otherwise healthy with no emotional or behavioural problems. His sister had walked in her sleep a few times between the ages of 6 and 9, and his father had had similar episodes when he was a child, but these had stopped in his teens.

The GP made a diagnosis of sleep terrors and explained that this, and the related condition of sleepwalking, were not uncommon in children, often ran in families, and almost always stopped after just a few years at most.

His parents were reassured that, although Sam seemed distressed during these episodes, this was not the case because he was still asleep at the time. They were advised not to try to wake him up, which would be difficult and would frighten him, even if they succeeded.

It was recommended that Sam should avoid becoming overtired as this could bring on an attack. Just for the duration of the school outing, Sam was prescribed a small bedtime dose of a benzodiazepine. His condition and its treatment were explained to the teachers who accompanied the children on the trip, which passed without incident.

Two years later, the episodes had stopped completely.

## Parasomnias later in the night in REM (dreaming) sleep

As described previously (see Figure 3.1), the last third of the night is when most REM sleep occurs. Therefore, parasomnias that are linked mainly to this form of sleep are most likely to occur later in the night. Remember that dreaming occurs mainly in REM sleep.

### Nightmares

These are dreams that are so frightening that they wake you up (as distinct from disturbing dreams without waking). They are the best known of the dramatic REM parasomnias. The term 'nightmare' is sometimes loosely used to refer to any seemingly frightening experience at night, such as agitated sleep-walking or sleep terrors (see earlier this chapter). In fact, true nightmares are a very different condition.

Typically, someone having a nightmare wakes up later in the night, alarmed and fully alert, and able to describe having just had a frightening vividly recalled dream often involving himself. He can be comforted and eventually will calm down and go back to sleep.

Occasional true nightmares are common, especially in children. They can be considered normal, often occurring for no obvious reason (although they may follow a frightening television programme before bedtime or some other alarming everyday experience) and do not need to be treated. However, if they are frequent or particularly distressing, you need to seek treatment for the underlying cause. This may be a significant emotional upset. Frequent distressing nightmares are often part of post-traumatic stress disorder following any sort of intensely distressing experience. In these circumstances, the content of the nightmares may indicate the original cause of distress.

A number of possible psychological treatments can be used (with professional advice) such as practising going over the contents of the nightmare (if consistent) but changing the end to something less frightening. More general psychiatric help may also be required.

## Case study

### Nightmares

James, a 24-year-old man, had been perfectly well with no sleep problems until soon after his sister, to whom he was very close, was killed in a road traffic accident. He had been in the passenger seat of the car that she was driving. At least once a week, he began to wake up later in the night in a highly distressed state, weeping profusely. Each time he described having had the same sort of dream in which he had relived the circumstances of the accident.

His girlfriend described how, during these dream experiences, he became increasingly restless in his sleep to the extent that she was woken up. Then James himself suddenly woke up shouting out his sister's name, even though he seemed fully alert and aware of where he was.

She was able to comfort him with reassurances that he had been having a 'bad dream', although it could take up to 15 minutes or so before he was able to calm down enough to get back to sleep.

It was obvious what had brought on the nightmares. The family doctor's advice was to vent his feelings about his sister's death by talking with his girlfriend and members of his family to see if the nightmares became less frequent with time. He hesitated to prescribe any medication at that stage, but arranged to see him every fortnight or so.

No real progress was made in the following few weeks. In fact, matters worsened. James remained grief-stricken and had become generally depressed. He was now reliving the accident repeatedly, not only in his nightmares but also during the day, and was pre-occupied with the details, despite trying to think of other things in order to distract himself.

He was tempted to try to ease his distress by drinking, but had resisted doing so, if only for his girlfriend's sake.

The doctor referred him to the local psychiatric services where he was considered to need fairly intensive treatment as an outpatient for his developing symptoms of post-traumatic stress disorder. Over the next few months, with a combination of bereavement counselling, a brief course of cognitive–behavioural therapy (see Chapter 8) and antidepressant treatment (a 'selective serotonin re-uptake inhibitor' drug), he gradually got better with a significant reduction in the frequency and intensity of his nightmares.

**Table 10.1** Comparison of arousal disorders and nightmares

| Arousal disorders | Nightmares |
|---|---|
| Common. | Common. |
| Family history usual. | No family history. |
| Occur in first third of the night (from SWS). | Occur late in the night (in REM sleep). |
| Risk of injury. | Injury unlikely. |
| Often dramatic. | Distressed and fully woken by frightening dream. |
| Person is asleep at the time and is therefore inaccessible and cannot be comforted (sometimes waking at the end). | Person is accessible on waking, needs comforting, and takes a while to calm down. |
| No memory of events. | Dream vividly recalled. |
| If awoken, the person is confused and possibly frightened. | Alarmed on waking. |
| Variable frequency and duration. | If frequent, there may be an underlying emotional disorder. |
| Usually no medical or psychiatric disorder. | Underlying disorder if frequent and severe. |
| Mostly cease spontaneously in time. | Usually temporary. |

As mentioned above, nightmares are sometimes confused with arousal disorders (and indeed other parasomnias) because of the inaccurate use of the term 'nightmare'. Table 10.1 sets out the main contrasting features of these two types of parasomnia, which are important to distinguish from each other because they are so different in their significance and advice and treatment requirements.

## REM sleep behaviour disorder

Another less common type of parasomnia occurs when people (usually elderly men, but also some women and occasionally children) are able to move during REM sleep, which is not normally possible (see Chapter 3). This makes them capable of acting out their dreams. If the dream is violent, they may injure themselves or others nearby by violent movements or actions while still asleep such as dramatic arm movements, punching, kicking, leaping, or running about. Much noise may accompany this behaviour, which is usually out of character for the person in question. This condition is called REM sleep behaviour disorder (RBD).

In some cases, the cause is not clear (so-called 'idiopathic RBD'). However, it is now known quite often to be a sign of neurological conditions such as Parkinson's disease and some forms of dementia, or other sleep disorders such as narcolepsy. It has also occasionally been linked to certain types of medication including some antidepressants.

Where the cause can be identified, the term 'symptomatic RBD' is used. Sometimes, the RBD precedes (perhaps by several years) the development of more precise signs of the underlying condition. Once recognized, RBD is usually easily treated, mainly by means of the benzodiazepine drug clonazepam.

Occasionally, RBD occurs in combination with an arousal disorder (see earlier this chapter). This is call 'parasomnia overlap disorder'.

---

## 🗎 Case study

### REM sleep behaviour disorder

The wife of Martin, aged 66, was alarmed about her husband's increasingly violent behaviour at night over the previous 2 years. She described how, while asleep, Martin shouted or screamed and sometimes dived out of bed. At times, he had punched and attacked her or gripped her tightly round the head or neck. He would then wake up and say that he had just had a dream in which he was fighting someone or trying to escape from danger. For the last few months, he had generally been irritable and easily distressed during the day and more than usually forgetful.

The couple had been happily married for 43 years. Martin had always been a mild-mannered man who lived a quiet life. He did not smoke or drink. His general health had been good and he had not experienced any other problems with his sleep. No one else in the family had a sleep problem.

The GP referred Martin to a local sleep disorders clinic. There was no sign of any neurological or other medical disorder and his mental state was considered normal apart from his memory, which, on testing, was borderline normal for his age. The results of sleep recordings, including audio-visual monitoring overnight in hospital (during which Martin had one of his violent episodes) were consistent with a diagnosis of RBD. In particular, his muscles were not inactive during REM sleep (in contrast to the normal finding of muscular paralysis during this type of sleep), allowing him to act out his dreams.

Martin was prescribed clonazepam, which stopped the violent episodes. He is being reviewed at intervals, as RBD can be an early sign of other neurological conditions.

### Groaning during sleep

This recently described parasomnia occurs mainly in REM sleep later in the night. It appears to be quite rare. Often it begins in childhood. It may well occur every night and disturb anyone sleeping nearby. Typically, breathing slows down and then, associated with breathing out (in contrast to obstructive sleep apnoea), a loud groan or moan (or possibly another strange noise) is emitted without the person waking up or any other change taking place. The groaning stops with a change of position in bed, but is then likely to start up again. The episodes tend to occur in clusters, each lasting a variable period. There is no known effective treatment.

## Parasomnias when waking up

As mentioned earlier, hypnopompic hallucinations and sleep paralysis are related to the process of awakening.

# Parasomnias at various times of the night

## Sleeptalking

Sleeptalking (either muttering or having limited conversations) is very common. It can occur by itself or in normal dreams, nightmares, sleepwalking, or RBD. Usually, in itself, talking in your sleep requires no treatment, but correction of any associated sleep disorder is required.

## Bedwetting ('nocturnal enuresis')

This normally affects children, in whom the problem may be 'primary' (i.e. they have never been able to control their bladder, often because of delayed maturation of their bladder mechanisms) or 'secondary' (i.e. bladder control has been lost after initially acquiring control).

By definition, therefore, enuresis starting in adult life (affecting possibly 1–2% of the population) is secondary, caused by conditions such as:

- urinary tract infection (especially in women);

- type 2 diabetes, starting later in life;

- prostate problems;

- obstructive sleep apnoea; and

- nocturnal epilepsy or some other neurological disorder.

Obviously, the cause of nocturnal enuresis in an adult needs to be considered carefully by your doctor.

## Frequently occurring arousal disorder episodes

These can also occur at any time during the night, although, as mentioned earlier in this chapter, such episodes usually occur early in the night.

## Various other medical or psychiatric conditions (and their treatments)

These can cause episodes of distressed or disturbed behaviour at night, the timing of which (collectively) can be variable. As emphasized previously, this is not often the cause of a parasomnia compared with other possible explanations. These episodes due to other conditions are called 'secondary parasomnias'.

Sometimes certain medications induce parasomnias. For example, some drugs used to treat high blood pressure and others for Parkinson's disease can cause nightmares and vivid dreams. Some antidepressants have been linked to sleep-walking, periodic limb movements, and RBD (see earlier this chapter).

The following are the main examples. Each tends to have its own distinctive features, which are recognizable by means of careful assessment, often including special recordings. Treatment varies widely, depending on the condition.

## Medical parasomnias

In certain types of epilepsy, the seizures occur mainly or always during sleep. Often, the seizures take the form of unusual behaviour or strange experiences (rather than convulsions) and may be similar to those in non-epileptic para-somnias (such as sleep terrors), which generally are much more common. Some of these epilepsies stop eventually of their own accord, while others need treatment based on the underlying cause.

Some types of headache can begin during sleep and cause strange or distressing experiences. These include certain forms of migraine and 'cluster headaches' (both of which can also occur during the day) and 'hypnic headaches', so called because they only occur during sleep. OSA can also cause headaches, both during sleep and on waking next morning.

Waking up in a frightened state because of difficulty breathing can occur in OSA and asthma.

People with gastrointestinal problems such as heartburn from gastro-oesophageal reflux or peptic ulcer pain may also wake in the night in a distressed state. Angina from coronary artery disease, with its characteristic sensation of chest pressure or pain, can also occur at night.

As mentioned elsewhere, restless legs syndrome (see Chapter 7) and periodic limb movements in sleep (see Chapter 9) can be symptoms of a medical disorder. RBD is also often associated with neurological disease and sometimes with medication.

---

📄 Case study

### Night-time epileptic attacks

For some years, Jane, a 20-year-old woman, had been having episodes of strange behaviour on average once a fortnight, mainly at various times of night but also occasionally during the day. Despite the daytime events, she had been diagnosed as having 'nightmares'. No particular advice or treatment had been provided in the hope that the episodes would gradually stop.

As this had not happened and showed no signs of doing so, she was eventually referred to a neurology clinic where the diagnosis of nightmares was thought unlikely in view of the fact that the episodes showed none of the characteristic features of that condition (see earlier this chapter). Other possibilities were considered, including the types of epilepsy known to be closely linked to sleep.

A detailed assessment of Jane's physical and mental condition revealed no abnormalities. In particular, there were no signs of neurological abnormality on examination or from brain-imaging studies. No one else in the family had this or any similar sort of complaint.

She was then admitted to the hospital for long-term monitoring of her episodes. This included several days of continuous recording of her brain activity by electroencephalogram (EEG), together with audio-visual monitoring, in the hope of capturing one or more of the episodes. Fortunately, this proved possible and showed consistent findings.

Each episode began with a sudden apparent awakening or, in the one daytime attack recorded, abrupt interruption of what she was doing at the time. This was immediately followed by rocking, kicking, and thrashing movements, accompanied by grunting and moaning sounds. After approximately a minute at most, her body stiffened all over before she let out a loud shout, whereupon the episode stopped abruptly and she became her normal self again. During each attack, she showed no response to being spoken to and seemed generally unaware of her surroundings.

The recording at the start of each attack clearly showed an abnormal electrical discharge starting in the frontal part of the brain on the right-hand side and spreading over a wider area mainly on the same side. On the basis of the nature of the attacks (very different from most other types of epilepsy) and the accompanying EEG findings (which are not always as clear-cut as this), a diagnosis of 'nocturnal frontal lobe epilepsy' was made, the cause of which was not apparent. Treatment with anti-epileptic medication was started and, with some later adjustments to the dose, after about 8 weeks the seizures stopped both at night and during the day.

## Psychiatric parasomnias

Again, recognition and treatment of the following examples require careful assessment and, possibly, hospital investigation.

- Reference has already been made earlier in this chapter to nightmares as a prominent feature of post-traumatic stress disorder.

- Nocturnal panic attacks, usually but not always accompanied by other such attacks during the day, share some features with other causes of fearful behaviour at night. However, the characteristic sign is that of an intense fear of 'impending doom', i.e. of imminent death. Various ways of reducing anxiety, including behavioural treatment or medication, can be helpful.

- Sleep-related eating disorder is mainly a problem in women who may or may not have an eating disorder that also affects them during the day. The night-time behaviour can be linked to other sleep disorders (mainly sleep-walking but sometimes OSA or narcolepsy, for example), in which case treatment is for the associated sleep disorder.

- In so-called 'dissociative states', people behave in ways in which, for psychological reasons, they are seemingly unaware. Sometimes this takes the form of dramatic behaviour at night while they are awake.

As far as possible, this last condition needs to be distinguished from malingering where someone behaves in strange ways at night but is fully aware of what they are doing and why, for example to gain attention or sympathy. Clearly, in both dissociative states and malingering the reason for behaving in these ways needs to be determined so that appropriate help can be provided.

## Case study

### Panic attacks

Alan, a 35-year-old man, went on a business trip to the Far East. The outward flight from the UK was considerably delayed and, after the long flight during which he was unable to sleep, he eventually arrived at his stop-over hotel in the early hours of the morning with the intention of undertaking the next stage of the journey the following day.

He went to bed in the hope of getting a few hours sleep but soon woke up in a fearful state, initially not knowing where he was, sweating and his heart pounding with a tight feeling in his chest, breathing heavily and trembling all over. He felt totally out of control and was convinced that he might be having a heart attack.

His first thought was to escape but, in the circumstances, he did not know where to go. He found the number for the hotel's emergency doctor but could not get a reply, which made him feel worse. Having decided that he would have to abandon the whole trip, he then rang the office of the airline with which he had flown to his present destination to find out the time of the next flight home.

For want of a better idea, Alan drank some beer from the mini-bar in the hope that it would settle him. This seemed to work after 10 minutes or so, and he went back to sleep for about 2 hours, only to wake up again in the same fearful state. This lasted for about the same length of time before he began to sleep fitfully again.

In fact, this sort of thing had happened to him before but almost always during the day, sometimes in stressful situations but at other times for no apparent reason. On this occasion, he readily recognized that he had experienced further 'panic attacks' (which he had read about), but knowing this did nothing to quieten his anxiety.

By breakfast time, he had recovered his composure enough to continue with his journey as originally planned, which he managed to do successfully, although he was somewhat apprehensive that this distressing experience might recur at any time.

When Alan returned home, he consulted his family doctor, who explained that panic attacks are quite common, although somewhat unusual at night. In his case, of the many possible causes and triggers, they were likely to be due to an inherited tendency (other members of the family had the same problem) and precipitated on this occasion by a combination of sleep loss and concern about the outcome of the important business venture involved.

Various treatment options were discussed, including cognitive–behavioural therapy (see Chapter 8) and anti-anxiety medication if the attacks were particularly troublesome. Breathing into a paper bag (to correct the imbalance of oxygen and carbon dioxide in the blood caused by rapid breathing or breathing too deeply in a panic attack) was mentioned as a possible useful remedy to help settle himself in the future, rather than using alcohol.

# 11

# Particular groups at special risk of sleep problems and their consequences

## ➔ Key points

◆ Sleep problems can affect anyone, but certain groups of people, for particular reasons, are at special risk of disturbed sleep and its harmful effects.

◆ Parents' sleep may well suffer if their child's sleep is a problem. The nature of their child's sleep disturbance, and ways in which it can be prevented or treated, vary with the child's stage of development.

◆ Women may suffer sleeping difficulties related to pregnancy, menstruation, child care, and the menopause, but can often be helped during these times. Your bed partner's own sleep disorder can also seriously disturb your sleep.

◆ Sleep problems are particularly common in elderly people, often because of a combination of social, medical, and psychiatric factors, although these can normally be corrected to some extent. Sleeping tablets are particularly hazardous at this age.

◆ Profound changes in sleep patterns often occur in people with dementia, causing much difficulty for carers.

◆ People with a learning disability are also particularly prone to sleep disorders, but such problems can frequently be treated effectively,

> mainly by behavioural methods but sometimes by medical intervention, depending on the cause.
>
> ◆ The common problems of shift workers can sometimes be reduced by alterations in shift-work patterns and other means.
>
> ◆ Various measures can be helpful to long-distance travellers subject to jet lag.
>
> ◆ Important precautions should be taken by drivers to prevent accidents caused by tiredness.

Groups of people who are particularly predisposed to sleep problems of one sort or another have been mentioned previously at various points in the book. This chapter provides further details on certain 'high-risk' members of the community.

## Parents

> ❌ Myth versus fact
>
> ❌ **Myth**: Having children inevitably means that you have a bad time through loss of sleep.
>
> ❗ **Fact**: Actually, children's sleep problems can usually be avoided or helped, and their parents' sleep protected, if appropriate advice or treatment is provided.

### Babies

Many parents of new babies lose sleep from having to attend to their baby's needs at night. Contrary to what is often supposed, this does not have to go on for very long. By 6 months or so, a baby's body clock has developed enough for feeding to be confined to the daytime after night-time feeds have gradually been withdrawn.

Also, the risk of later sleep problems can be reduced by teaching your child good sleep habits from very early on. Basic ways of doing this include:

◆ establishing a consistent 24-hour routine for your baby including a progressively calming sequence of events as bedtime approaches; and

◆ creating a clear difference between your baby's daytime and night-time experiences in order to promote the development of his circadian sleep–wake rhythm.

For further details of children's sleep problems from babyhood to adolescence, see Sources of further information in the Appendix.

## Toddlers

A quarter or more of children between the ages of 1 and 3 have troublesome sleep problems. Many parents of toddlers are only too familiar with bedtime difficulties that cause much distress to all concerned. The situation is made worse if their child also wakes in the night demanding their attention.

The relationship between you and your child is likely to be affected, and your well-being and ability to cope at home or work impaired, if you persistently lose sleep in this way. If sleep problems have already become established, they can be corrected as follows:

◆ Introduce a consistent evening routine, resulting in your child being relaxed and ready to sleep at bedtime.

◆ Be firm, if necessary, about difficult behaviour at bedtime ('setting limits') without issuing threats.

◆ Avoid reinforcement of problem behaviour by giving too much attention to it.

◆ Make the bedroom a relaxed place to sleep rather than somewhere to play, get excited, or be punished.

◆ For most families, encourage the child to go to sleep in his own bed and without you, so that if he wakes in the night he can go back to sleep on his own.

This last point is also important for preventing sleep problems.

Putting these measures into practice might need the help of an experienced health visitor or psychologist. Sleeping medicine is generally inadvisable. Often, it does not work and can lead to your child being drowsy or irritable during the day.

## 📄 Case study

### Sleeplessness in a young child

Andy, a healthy 4-year-old, was very distressed at bedtime unless one of his parents (usually his mother) was in his room with him until he fell asleep. When he woke at night, he again wanted someone with him or insisted on joining his parents in their bed.

This had been a problem for as long as they could remember, but it had become particularly troublesome, especially for his mother, who complained that she constantly felt tired and stressed, particularly since the arrival of a new baby. Sleeping medicine for Andy had not worked.

The family doctor put the parents in touch with a psychologist at the local children's hospital who suggested that mother and, when available, father (who often worked away from home) should deal with the bedtime problem by teaching Andy to fall asleep by himself.

This was achieved by gradually removing themselves from being with him in his bedroom, sitting progressively further away from him until they were outside the room. They were told to interact with Andy as little as possible while this was going on.

His parents persisted with this procedure, even though initially he cried out for them. To their delight, after a week he was able to settle to sleep without them. As he had learned to go to sleep at bedtime by himself, he also became able to settle himself back to sleep when he woke in the night.

From then on, Andy's sleep was not a problem. His mother in particular felt very much better as a result of consistently being able to obtain a good night's sleep.

### Older children

The sleeplessness problems just discussed can persist in older (pre-pubertal) children if not dealt with adequately. However, at this age the pattern of sleep problems tends to have changed and affects parents' sleep in different ways:

◆ Difficulty getting off to sleep may still be an issue but is more likely to be caused by being over-aroused at bedtime because of boisterous activities, exciting or frightening stories or television programmes, or other inappropriate stimulating bedroom activities, all of which are best discouraged.

◆ Night-time fears become more likely at this stage and may need special attention, depending on their nature and severity.

◆ Stress, worry, or upset about family or school issues are also a possible cause of troubled sleep.

◆ It is important that bedtime is not set so early that your child is not yet ready to sleep (see the 'forbidden zone', Chapter 3).

◆ Arousal disorders, bedwetting, and some other parasomnias (see Chapter 10) are also common at this age.

## Adolescents

The biological body clock changes that occur at puberty, and adolescents' sleep requirements, are discussed in Chapter 4. Combined with life-style changes, inadequate sleep and its consequences are a common problem at this age, often resulting in delayed sleep-phase syndrome (see Chapters 7 and 9).

Partly because of misinterpretation of the true situation (see Chapter 12), this can easily cause much parental concern and adverse effects on their sleep. This difficult and a possibly fraught situation at home can be made worse by parents losing sleep waiting anxiously for their teenager's return home from late-night social activities.

# Women

## ❌ Myth versus fact

❌ **Myth**: Women just worry a lot. That's why they don't sleep as well as men.

❶ **Fact**: This may be true in some cases. However, there are other quite different possibilities that need to be considered and dealt with if necessary.

Women are predisposed to sleep problems in various special ways, as described in the box below, for which there may not be a counterpart in men.

# Possible causes of women's sleep problems

## Pregnancy

- Excessive tiredness caused by increased physical demands.

- Physical discomfort—especially in later stages.

- Anxiety about pregnancy and motherhood.

- Post-partum changes.

## Menstrual cycle

- Insomnia from pre-menstrual tension or depression.

- Excessive sleepiness during the pre-menstrual period.

- Sleep disturbance as part of dysmenorrhoea.

## Child care

- Babies' night-time feeding.

- Sleep problems in toddlers.

- A disabled or chronically ill child.

## Other caring roles

- Elderly family members (including those suffering from dementia).

## Menopause

- Hormonal changes.

## Bed partner

- Snoring, jerking limbs, or restlessness.

## Pregnancy

An increased need to sleep is common in the first few weeks of pregnancy after which the problem usually disappears. During the later stages of pregnancy, it might be increasingly difficult to get off to sleep or stay asleep as a result of leg cramps, backache, or other physical discomfort as the fetus grows larger.

There are additional ways in which sleep can be disturbed:

- Periodic limb movements (see Chapter 9) and sleep-related breathing problems can occur or worsen during pregnancy.

- Anxiety about being pregnant and impending motherhood can also disturb sleep, sometimes producing frightening dreams.

If you consult your doctor, he will need to know if the sleep problems are new and so can be attributed to your being pregnant or whether there was a pre-existing sleep disorder that might have been made worse by your pregnancy. Whenever possible, medication, including sleeping tablets, should be avoided during pregnancy.

In most cases where your sleep has been disturbed by being pregnant, you can be reassured that things will improve after the birth and you will not need drug treatment, especially if you follow sleep hygiene guidelines (see Chapter 8), with the help of your partner, if necessary. A possible exception is that post-partum changes in mood and general well-being can interfere with sleep, in which case help specifically with these aspects will be required.

## Menstrual cycle

Disturbed sleep can be related to the menstrual cycle in a number of ways:

- Pre-menstrual tension or depression can be accompanied by insomnia or excessive sleepiness.

- Some women become sleepy in the first few days of their period. A hormonal explanation seems likely because, in severe cases, treatment with an oral contraceptive has sometimes been helpful.

- Sleep can be disturbed by painful menstrual cramps ('dysmenorrhoea').

## Child care

Mothers in particular lose sleep by having to attend to their infants at night. However, babies are usually capable of doing without night-time feeds by about 6 months of age, as discussed earlier in this chapter. In the meantime, interaction with the baby during feeds at night is best kept to a minimum and bright lights should be avoided.

It is mainly mothers whose sleep is disturbed by toddlers who wake in the night demanding their parents' attention. This common problem (often accompanied by bedtime difficulties) can usually be avoided or treated by teaching children good sleep habits and encouraging them to go to sleep without their parents being with them. Again, the care (by day and night) of disabled or chronically ill children usually falls mainly to mothers.

### Other caring roles

For the most part, women have the main responsibility for caring for ageing family members, including those with dementia whose particularly severe sleep disturbance is discussed below. This often causes disruption of carers' own sleep patterns to a serious degree, with inevitable adverse consequences.

### Menopause

Women who are troubled by insomnia, often accompanied by night sweats and hot flushes, during the menopause might be helped by hormone replacement therapy. However, this requires careful medical supervision in view of concerns about possible harmful effects. Sleep problems caused by depression can also occur at this time of life.

### Bed partners

A bed partner who snores (see Chapter 9), groans, has jerky limb movements, or is otherwise restless at night (see Chapter 10) can seriously disrupt your sleep.

## Elderly people

> ### ❌ Myth versus fact
>
> ❌ **Myth**: Poor sleep cannot be avoided when you are old.
>
> ❗ **Fact**: This is not so. Whatever your age, something can usually be done to help you sleep better when the cause of your sleep problem is identified.

By recalling the times that they are awake and misinterpreting these awakenings as abnormal, some elderly people (and indeed others) underestimate how much they sleep at night and become worried and need reassurance that their sleep is actually within normal limits. This is one aspect of 'sleep education' (see Chapter 8).

## Causes of sleep problems in later life

The various changes in sleep patterns that are associated with later life (see Chapter 4) combine to make genuinely unsatisfactory sleep particularly common. The main sleep complaints expressed by older people are about insomnia, the various forms of which are described in Chapter 7.

The problem is made worse if you have a medical condition or psychological problems (such as those related to bereavement, loneliness, or financial difficulties), which themselves interfere with sleep. Waking frequently at night to empty your bladder (because of a prostate problem, for example) is a common cause of disrupted sleep in elderly people. Also, certain sleep disorders that can impair the quality of sleep—such as obstructive sleep apnoea (OSA) and periodic limb movements in sleep; see Chapter 9—appear to occur more often in the elderly.

Family members or care staff in hospitals or nursing homes may also notice unusual sleep patterns, including mistiming of the sleep period or disturbed behaviour at night.

## Prevention and treatment

It should not be assumed that poor sleep is an inevitable part of getting older. Accurate diagnosis of the cause(s) (which may be multiple) and the correct treatment or a change in lifestyle can improve sleep.

It is obviously important that underlying medical or psychiatric disorders affecting sleep should be treated effectively. Doctors must also make sure that any medications prescribed for such disorders do not themselves interfere with sleep. If they do, an alternative treatment should be prescribed if possible. It is important to ensure good sleep hygiene and to keep socially active and generally fit—for example, by taking regular, mild outdoor exercise. A short afternoon nap can be beneficial, but sleeping for longer than 20 minutes in the daytime can make it more difficult to sleep at night (see Chapter 3).

## Special precautions

Sleeping tablets are usually not a good idea at any age (see Chapter 8), despite often being prescribed. This is especially so in later life when it is easy to take too high a dose for the body to cope with. This is likely to cause excessive sleepiness during the day, confusion, unsteadiness, and possible injury from falls. They can also cause problems by interacting with other medications or with alcohol.

As mentioned earlier, some sleeping tablets can worsen breathing problems during sleep (including OSA). At best, a very short course of sleeping tablets might be justified for someone who is particularly distressed by not sleeping well, but only while the cause of the sleep problem is being assessed before appropriate treatment is decided upon.

Anyone who has been taking sleeping tablets for a long time may experience unpleasant withdrawal effects (see Chapter 8) if they stop taking them suddenly because the body will have become used to the drug being in their system. This danger applies particularly in the elderly. The medication should be reduced gradually under the guidance of a doctor experienced in such matters.

Over-the-counter medications, and medicines belonging to other people, should not be used to improve sleep. An exception to these restraints on using medication in elderly people is the use of clonazepam for REM sleep behaviour disorder (see Chapter 10), which occurs mainly in elderly men.

### Case study

#### Insomnia in an elderly person

Ted, a 73-year-old man, complained to his GP that for some years he had hardly slept at all. He also described a distressing feeling of ill-defined discomfort and agitation in his legs that came on in the late evening. This was worse when he lay down in bed at night or when he woke up at night, which he did frequently to pass water. To try to get some relief, he would rub his legs vigorously or walk around the room, sometimes for long periods.

In addition, he complained of painful joints, which also made it difficult to sleep. Ted's wife (whose own sleep was seriously disturbed as a result of her husband's sleep problems) described frequent jerking of his legs when he was asleep. She said that he was always dozing off during the day and had little enthusiasm for the things that used to interest him.

The GP felt that there was no convincing evidence of sleep apnoea and that, despite the sleep problems, Ted was not depressed. The only main finding on physical examination was an enlarged prostate, which probably accounted for his frequent visits to the toilet at night. He was referred to a urologist for this.

A combination of medication for his restless legs syndrome (see Chapter 7) and periodic limb movements (see Chapter 9), which were confirmed by polysomnography, and analgesics for his joint pains, together with sleep hygiene advice (especially about not sleeping much, if at all, during the day) led to a significant improvement in Ted's sleep and general well-being. Treatment for his urinary problems is still being considered.

## People with dementia

 Myth versus fact

❌ **Myth**: Nothing can be done to help someone with dementia to sleep better.

❗ **Fact**: Treatment can be difficult but, depending on the cause, some improvement may be possible.

Sleep disturbance in people with dementia can be a serious problem and a particular challenge for carers at home, in hospital, or in a care home. Apart from the changes to be expected as part of the ageing process (see Chapter 4), much more severe disruption of sleep often occurs, including restlessness, wandering, confusion, and agitation at night, with very irregular sleep patterns throughout the 24-hour period.

Treating such problems can be very difficult. Excessive medication is likely to make the problems worse, although some form of sedation may be necessary. As far as possible, the sleep hygiene principles explained in Chapter 8 should be encouraged, including regular exposure to sunlight, which can help to re-establish a more normal sleep–wake rhythm.

More research is needed on the best way of combating this difficult problem including, for example, the possible use of melatonin.

## 📄 Case study

### Dementia

Christine, a middle-aged unmarried woman, visited her GP complaining that she felt constantly tired and exhausted. It soon came to light that, for the last 3 years, she had single-handedly been looking after her aged widowed father who had been diagnosed as suffering from quite severe Alzheimer's disease.

Over that time, her father's sleep had become progressively more disturbed with the result that Christine's own sleep had suffered badly. This had added significantly to the difficulties of providing the constant care and attention that he needed.

The main problem was that Christine's father hardly slept at all at night which he mostly spent in an agitated, restless state, wandering about in a confused fashion. During the day, he slept for long periods, making it difficult to feed him at appropriate times and to attend to his other basic needs. Attempts to do so were met with resistance and even aggression. As it was no longer possible for him to be taken out during the daytime, the two of them were essentially housebound.

Once the GP realized the magnitude of these problems, he sought the advice of the local psychogeriatric unit and admission for assessment was arranged. With the help of a sleep disorders clinic, it was possible to exclude physical factors (other than the dementia), depression, and additional sleep disorders as complicating influences. The main emphasis, therefore, was placed on the difficult task of treating the sleep disorder itself.

It was thought appropriate to assess the effect of a more structured day–night routine, regular mild physical exercise, and other sleep hygiene measures. In addition, daily exposure to sunlight and restriction of exposure to light at night were recommended, intended to improve the patient's circadian sleep–wake rhythm. Medication was not thought likely to be helpful.

However, as there were no other family members to help Christine, and local home-nursing services were severely stretched, implementation of such measures was clearly beyond the daughter's resources and admission to a residential care home was organized with continued advice and support for the staff there.

This approach eventually proved successful to some extent and Christine, whose health and general well-being had improved significantly, was able to visit her father regularly.

# People with a learning disability (mental handicap)

> ## ❌ Myth versus fact
>
> ❌ **Myth**: You cannot expect someone with a learning disability to sleep well. They just can't learn how to do it.
>
> ❗ **Fact**: The same basic principles of teaching good sleep habits or treating sleep disorders that apply in other people often work.

Sleep disorders are particularly common in children and adults with a learning disability. Because of sleep loss or poor-quality sleep, they can increase the daytime problems of learning and behaviour and add significantly to the difficulties of carers.

Sleep problems are often the result of not learning good sleep habits, but physical factors can also be important such as OSA in Down syndrome and many other causes of learning disability. Associated neurological conditions, such as epilepsy or autism, can disrupt sleep further.

As in other groups, careful attention should routinely be paid by doctors to the possible presence, causes, and consequences for the individual and their family of the sleep disorder. Psychologists should also be well placed to explore these aspects, and, where appropriate, to carry out treatment of a psychological type, which can be very effective, even if the sleep problem has been severe and long-standing.

> ## 📄 Case study
>
> ### Sleep problems and learning disability
>
> The parents of Chrissie, a 16-year-old girl with Down syndrome and quite a severe learning disability, reported that she had never slept well for as long as they could remember, waking repeatedly in the night, sometimes for long periods. When this happened, she insisted on joining them in their bed.
>
> They had tried sleeping medicine in the past but it had not worked and seemed to make Chrissie drowsy during the day. Eventually, they tried to reconcile themselves to the idea that such problems were inevitable in

someone with a learning disability and that nothing could be done. For want of a better idea, they had continued to let her sleep in their bed. However, the sleep problem had become worse and, as Chrissie became older and bigger, the parents became particularly worried at the prospect of her wanting to sleep with them indefinitely. They were also worried that she had steadily become more irritable and easily upset at home and at school.

They talked about their increasing concerns to their GP, who referred them to a sleep disorders clinic. When a full sleep history was taken there, it was revealed that, in addition to the settling and night-waking problems, Chrissie was very restless when asleep and repeatedly stopped breathing for many seconds, making gasping and choking noises at the end of each pause.

It was explained to the parents that these findings were highly suggestive of OSA, which is very common in people with Down syndrome because their upper airway is narrower than normal and easily blocks off when they are asleep.

It was pointed out that treatment can be difficult, but that some people with Down syndrome benefit from removal of the tonsils and adenoids (which, even though they might not be particularly enlarged, can add to the risk of the airway being blocked). This possibility is being considered in the hope that Chrissie's sleep will become more settled and of better quality and that this might help to improve the way she feels and behaves during the day.

In the meantime, her parents were encouraged to return her to her own bed, gently but firmly, when she came into their room at night. To begin with, she objected loudly but they persisted, having been told that the situation might get worse before getting better. Over the next few nights, she gradually objected less. On the sixth night, she stayed in her room the whole time and has continued to do so, without any signs of distress.

Ideally, Chrissie's sleep problems should have been investigated and treated at a much earlier stage, saving her and her parents much trouble over the years. However, better late than never, and at least now their difficulties have been lessened, demonstrating that even simple behavioural treatments can rapidly be effective in severe and long-standing sleep problems, whatever the person's intellectual level.

# Shift workers

## ❌ Myth versus fact

❌ **Myth**: Someone who starts working night shifts will soon adjust and sleep perfectly well during the day instead of at night.

❗ **Fact**: Unfortunately, this is often not the case. Advice on working practices and help to minimize the effect of disrupted sleep are essential to prevent potentially serious consequences.

Many people now work what can be called anti-social hours, including working for very long periods at a time. This not only risks causing inadequate sleep and accumulating sleep debt with its adverse effects (see Chapter 2), but in the process also interferes with family and other aspects of social life.

Night-shift work has become commonplace, often with shifts changing at short or irregular intervals. This is partly because there has been an increase in services availability (the '24-hour society'), although night work has always been part of some jobs such as police work or nursing.

Changing from working during the day to working at night upsets your circadian rhythms, including your sleep–wake cycle (see Chapter 3), and causes problems while you are awake. It affects you in a similar way to jet lag (see below) but can be much more persistent and serious in its consequences.

The harmful effects are usually worse when you frequently change between day work and night work each week. This is because your body clock controlling the times of being awake and asleep does not have time to adjust to each new work pattern. However, even with longer shift rotations, many people (especially those over the age of 40) do not adapt well to night work. The problem is often complicated because people tend to revert to daytime activities at weekends or during the holidays to fit in with family life.

### Problems arising from shift work

Night-shift workers are affected by the fact that their body clock is telling them that they should be asleep when they are having to work. In addition, the sleep that they obtain during the day is often shorter than usual and of poor quality.

For various reasons, shift work suits some people, but many others have difficulty adjusting to working at night in particular. As well as sleep, other basic functions are affected, and the person often develops various psychological and physical complaints, such as gastrointestinal problems. A bad situation will be made worse by attempting to sleep during the day by using alcohol or long-term sleeping tablets, or by trying to stay alert at night by drinking lots of coffee. As well as your general standard of work being affected, accidents can occur because of poor concentration, sometimes with serious consequences.

The social consequences of working anti-social hours are also unwelcome to many shift workers. Normal family and social life can be disrupted, sometimes leading to marital and other family problems. For health reasons, some people are considered particularly unsuitable for working night shifts. Occupational health staff should advise them against such work and recommend alternative arrangements. This applies to anyone with a pre-existing sleep disturbance, a serious physical or psychological disorder, or a history of alcohol or drug abuse, or if you are pregnant, as complications are reported to be increased.

## Minimizing the harmful effects

Employers should be mindful of the hazards of shift work and make appropriate arrangements to ensure that the risks are minimized. This might include organizing changes in shifts that are the least disruptive to circadian rhythms. These include:

◆ longer stretches of night work and day work;

◆ changing shifts by rotating them forward in time (which helps your body clock to adjust better than backwards rotation);

◆ providing high-intensity lighting to help offset the tendency to sleep; and

◆ possibly encouraging short naps during the working period, if appropriate.

Special care should be taken if you have to drive home after working a night shift (see below for advice about driving when sleepy).

As the daytime sleep of night-shift workers tends to be shorter than usual and of poorer quality, circumstances at home should be as conducive to sleep as possible. This means:

◆ quiet surroundings (by arrangement with others at home and possibly the use of earplugs);

◆ no interruptions;

◆ a darkened bedroom; and

◆ the avoidance of caffeine-containing drinks 2–3 hours before going to bed.

It is best to avoid resorting to sleeping tablets to help you sleep during the day. Practising other aspects of good sleep hygiene (see Chapter 8) and keeping to regular sleep and meal times (to avoid your circadian rhythms becoming generally disorganized) is also important. Relaxing weekday routines at weekends is likely to disrupt your body clock's attempts to adjust. Healthy eating and regular exercise, as a means of maintaining good general health, are desirable. Mutually satisfactory arrangements should be made with other members of the family about the best opportunities for contact with them to avoid neglect of family life. Other social activities should also be maintained as far as possible.

# Jet lag

## ❌ Myth versus fact

❌ **Myth**: Alcohol can help offset the effects of jet lag.

❶ **Fact**: This is not true. In fact, alcohol tends to disrupt sleep later in the sleep period and can also delay the adjustment of your circadian sleep–wake cycle.

Jet lag is the particular form of sleep disturbance that you experience when you travel so fast across time zones ('transmeridian travel') that your body cannot adapt to the time change. The same thing happens to pilots and other staff on long-haul flights. Travelling between north and south does not give rise to such difficulties.

In jet lag, your sleep–wake rhythm and other bodily circadian rhythms, such as body temperature, get out of step with the 24-hour dark–light cycle (see Chapter 3). Thus, there is a mismatch between your body's internal clock and the external (or local) clock. The mismatch and resulting problems get worse the more time zones you cross. Your body's circadian rhythms remain on the time at which the journey started and only shift slowly (at different rates) to the time at your destination. For each hour of time difference, it takes about a day to adapt.

People differ somewhat in their susceptibility to jet lag but, generally, at your new destination, you may find it difficult to get to sleep at the new night-time and, during the new daytime, you feel sleepy and easily fatigued, prone to headaches, and somewhat confused, and you may perform poorly. Your digestion might be upset and you may feel irritable or depressed. These symptoms are usually worse if you are already short of sleep at the start of your journey.

Jet lag is usually more severe when travelling from west to east (for example, from the USA to the UK). Although we operate on the basis of a 24-hour day, our body clock is programmed to operate on a day that is somewhat longer than 24 hours (see Chapter 3) and, in flying west, we are able to extend our day more readily than reducing the hours of our day when we fly in an easterly direction.

If you will only be in the new time zone for 1 or 2 days, if you can, you might be better off sleeping and eating and undertaking other usual activities when you would normally be doing so at home. However, if you have to work on arrival, you need to be able to function well at your destination. There are a number of measures that can help, especially if your trip is a long one, although individuals differ in their need to do these things and in the benefit they derive from them.

## Advice for travel across many time zones

The value of the following advice will depend on the individual and the nature of your journey. The aim is to minimize the effects of jet lag and also to avoid sleep loss, as far as possible, in order to reduce the risk of insomnia and daytime sleepiness. It is advantageous to travel by day, whenever possible. Opinions about the usefulness of melatonin (see Chapter 8) for jet lag vary. Exposure to daylight and experience of darkness is what most influences your sleep–wake pattern. In general, good sleep hygiene (see Chapter 8) helps you to recover from jet lag.

### Before travelling

◆　Avoid becoming sleep-deprived before the journey.

◆　For several days beforehand, begin to shift the timing of your sleep and activity patterns to correspond to those of your destination. In particular, go to bed early and get up early if you will be travelling eastwards; go to sleep later for westward travel.

◆　For 1–2 days before you travel, taking a fast-release form of melatonin (as distinct from the sustained-release form, which acts over a longer period) in the early evening, or exposing yourself to bright light in the morning, might be helpful if your journey is going to be eastwards.

♦ Over the same period, melatonin early in the morning or bright light in the evening (and sun glasses in bright light in the morning) can be helpful for westward travel.

## During the journey

♦ Make yourself as comfortable as possible (first or business class is best!).

♦ Sleep as much as you can during an overnight flight and stay awake during a daytime flight.

♦ During the night, refuse interruptions for meals or entertainment (ear plugs and an eye mask can help) and avoid caffeine and alcohol.

♦ Drink lots of water to avoid becoming dehydrated.

♦ Possibly use a short-acting sleeping tablet (i.e. one that promotes sleep for just a few hours; see Chapter 8).

## On arrival at your destination

♦ Adopt the new time for sleeping, meals, exercise, and other activities, whatever the direction you have travelled.

♦ If possible, avoid having to work in the first 24 hours.

♦ Avoid driving long distances on your first day.

♦ Take key decisions at the times when your body clock expects you to be awake.

♦ Avoid naps when you arrive after travelling eastwards.

♦ Caffeine during the day for the first day or so after travelling westwards can help to combat sleepiness.

♦ A short-acting sleeping tablet for the first few nights may be useful.

♦ To help your body clock adjust to the new clock time, melatonin in the evening or bright light in the morning for the first 1–2 days might be justified after an eastward journey.

♦ For the same period, melatonin in the morning or bright light in the evening is sometimes helpful after flying west.

# Drivers

> ### ❌ Myth versus fact
>
> ❌ **Myth**: If you feel sleepy when driving, all you need to do is wind down the car window and turn up the radio.
>
> ❗ **Fact**: This will have a very limited effect in keeping you awake. You need to do much more than this to prevent yourself falling asleep at the wheel (see below).

Being sleepy while driving can be as dangerous as drinking alcohol and driving. It is thought that about 20% of road accidents are caused by people falling asleep at the wheel. These kinds of accidents are likely to be serious, because the drivers do not swerve or put on their brakes. Typically, in such accidents you run into the vehicle in front or unknowingly weave about the carriageway or drift off it. Train drivers run the same risks as drivers of cars or trucks.

## Situations where you are more likely to fall asleep at the wheel

Certain circumstances can make driving accidents more likely to occur, especially when they occur in combination, in particular:

◆ when you are short of sleep or your sleep has been disrupted, for example, by working shifts;

◆ during the early hours of the morning when your tendency to sleep is greatest (and also to a lesser extent in the early afternoon at the time of the post-lunch dip; see Chapter 3);

◆ after long periods of continuous driving;

◆ where the driving conditions are monotonous (as in motorway driving);

◆ when you are by yourself in the vehicle;

◆ when the inside of the vehicle is comfortable and warm;

◆ if you have consumed alcohol; and

◆ if you have a sleep disorder that itself causes excessive sleepiness (such as OSA).

## Warning signs

The most important warning sign when you are driving is your own awareness of being sleepy. The signs of this are:

- yawning frequently;

- having trouble keeping your eyes open or focusing your vision;

- your head dropping forward;

- drifting across the traffic lanes;

- not recalling the road for the last minute or so (caused by slipping in and out of 'microsleeps' in which events are not registered and, therefore, not recalled); and

- feeling the need to fight off sleep.

## How to avoid becoming sleepy while driving

- You should make every effort to avoid being over-tired before you set out. Do not drive if you have missed a lot of sleep the night before or for longer periods beforehand.

- As far as possible, avoid driving at the times of night or day when you are most likely to fall asleep at the wheel (i.e. in the early hours of the morning and early afternoon; see Chapter 3).

- Avoid alcohol and drugs with a sedative effect, as both greatly increase the risk of accidents from sleepiness.

## What to do if you feel sleepy while driving

It is essential to realize that you might fall asleep very rapidly without further warning. The following advice is aimed at preventing this happening.

- You must stop driving as soon as possible.

- Until you can find a suitable place to stop the car, open the window to allow cool air to blow on your face and turn up the radio or CD player (although this is not enough on its own to stop you falling asleep).

- When you stop, take a break for at least 30 minutes.

◆ Just taking a walk or some exercise during your break will not offset sleepiness for very long.

◆ You will get the most benefit from your break if you drink at least two cups of strong caffeinated coffee and then have a nap for about 20 minutes—any longer and you may feel groggy afterwards ('sleep inertia'). You should drink the coffee before your nap because it takes up to 30 minutes for coffee to have its alerting effect. Doing both of these things is much more effective than doing either one alone.

## Driving with a sleep disorder

If you have a sleep disorder that makes you excessively sleepy, such as OSA or narcolepsy, it is important that your doctor assesses your fitness to drive safely. Until this has been done, you should avoid driving.

If you suffer from such a condition, you have a duty to inform the Driver and Vehicle Licensing Agency (DVLA) and your insurance company. The likelihood of you having an accident and your response to treatment will determine whether you can have a driving licence and for how long, and also the need for periodic reassessment (see Useful addresses in the Appendix).

# 12

# Sleep disorders misinterpreted as other medical or psychological conditions

## ⮕ Key points

- The psychological effects of insufficient or poor-quality sleep, and also excessive sleepiness, are easily misinterpreted as something other than a sleep disturbance. This is likely to happen where knowledge about sleep and its disorders is lacking.

- Certain specific sleep disorders are at particular risk of being misunderstood in this way.

- Combinations of more than one sleep disorder are possible.

- Careful assessment is essential for correct interpretation and diagnosis leading to appropriate advice and treatment.

## ✖ Myth versus fact

✖ **Myth**: It is obvious if someone has a sleep problem—they are simply tired.

❗ **Fact**: Nothing so simple! Sleep can be disturbed in many ways and for many different reasons. Because this is generally not realized, many sleep disorders are not recognized for what they really are.

# Correctly identifying sleep disorders

At several points in this book, it has been mentioned that sleep disorders can mistakenly be thought to be some other type of condition and nothing particularly to do with sleep. This will happen if the person themselves or their relatives or friends giving advice (or professionals whom they consult for help) do not know enough about the many types of sleep disturbance and the various ways in which you can be affected.

This is such an important matter that it is worth saying a little more about it in this chapter. If mistakes of this sort are made, the situation is likely to become very confused or frustrating and clearly the person with the sleep disorder will not get the help needed.

## General aspects of the misinterpretation of sleep disorders

If, as a result of any of the sleep disorders discussed in this book, you persistently do not get enough sleep or the quality of your sleep is poor, the way that you feel and behave is likely to be affected in a number of unwelcome ways (see Chapter 2). Tiredness, fatigue, irritability, poor concentration, impaired performance (possibly causing accidents at work or elsewhere), and depression are common examples of this.

Excessive daytime sleepiness, whatever its cause of the many possibilities (see Chapter 9), is often misjudged as laziness, disinterest and daydreaming, lack of motivation, depression, intellectual inadequacy, or a number of other states of mind.

The paradoxical effect of inadequate sleep causing over-activity in children, in contrast to the reduction in activity in sleepy adults, has led to some of them being labelled as having attention-deficit hyperactivity disorder (ADHD) and inappropriately being prescribed stimulant drugs, instead of being treated for their sleep disorder (see Chapter 2). The same may also apply in some adults assumed to have ADHD.

These various incorrect interpretations that overlook the role of sleep disturbance will inevitably cause the problems to persist. It is a serious matter if it is not appreciated that improvements in your sleep (which are usually perfectly possible with the right advice and treatment) will make you feel and perform much better and improve the quality of your life.

# Misinterpretation of individual sleep disorders

The features of many individual sleep disorders are open to misinterpretations of a more specific nature. The following are examples of this.

## Sleep starts

As a result of their sudden and often dramatic nature, sleep starts—involving a sudden jerk or intense sensory experiences when going off to sleep (as described in Chapter 10)—may be thought to indicate something physically wrong, such as epilepsy or another neurological disorder. This is not the case.

## Sleep paralysis and sleep hallucinations

The same reassurance can be given about the common experience of sleep paralysis (other than that associated with narcolepsy; see Chapter 10), which can mistakenly be thought to be symptoms of a stroke. Sleep-related hallucinations (see Chapter 10) can be considered as essentially benign, despite their sometimes striking nature. This is again true of the especially dramatic combination of sleep paralysis and complex hallucinations, which, if misinterpreted, may well be viewed as a serious psychiatric disorder.

## Rhythmic movements related to sleep

Parents of the many young children who bang their heads or roll about rhythmically at night (see Chapter 10) can erroneously think that this is evidence of an emotional problem or perhaps some form of epilepsy.

## Night-shift work sleep disorder

As described in Chapter 11, night-shift workers are subject to inadequate and poor-quality daytime sleep, as well as various bodily complaints including gastrointestinal discomfort, all of which may be thought to be primarily medical in origin, rather than the result of disruption of normal sleep–wake patterns. The psychological effects mentioned earlier of inadequate or poor-quality sleep, compounded by the disruptive influences of shift work on family and social life, are commonplace in shift workers. These unfortunate consequences may overshadow and distract from the true origins of the shift worker's problems.

## Jet lag

The effects of jet lag (see Chapter 11) are usually short-lived, but travellers (or, indeed aircrew, if preventative measures are not taken) who frequently cross several time zones on each flight can develop chronic sleep disturbances that can have serious effects on mood and performance, the true cause of which may not be appreciated.

## Delayed sleep-phase syndrome

Difficulty getting to sleep and also waking up in the morning, as well as daytime sleepiness and sleeping in at the weekend, which characterize delayed sleep-phase syndrome (see Chapter 9), is easily misinterpreted as awkward, lazy, or irresponsible behaviour, malingering, school refusal in young people, or being work-shy. In fact, this state of affairs is the result of a combination of biological body clock and lifestyle changes. The risk of the fundamental problem not being recognized is increased if alcohol or sedative drugs are taken in an attempt to get to sleep, or stimulants are used to try and stay awake during the day.

## Advanced sleep-phase syndrome

Because of body clock changes that can occur in old age (see Chapter 4), in advanced sleep-phase syndrome there is a tendency to fall asleep earlier than when younger. This might cause you to wake early in the morning because, by that time, you have obtained as much sleep as you need. This should not be mistaken for the early morning wakening associated with depression where the total amount of sleep is reduced.

## Arousal disorders

Generally, it is not realized that complicated behaviour can occur while some-one remains asleep during the relatively common conditions of sleepwalking and other arousal disorders (see Chapter 10). One view is that these disorders involve disturbances in the more primitive parts of the brain, including those responsible for the basic physiological processes involved in fear, hunger, aggression, and sexual activity. This can give rise to behaviours that are highly likely to be misinterpreted.

Clearly, if it is not known that such complicated behaviours are compatible with still being asleep, it will mistakenly be assumed that the person was awake at the time and aware of what he was doing, and therefore responsible (perhaps legally) for what happened.

## Obstructive sleep apnoea (OSA)

In adults, OSA (see Chapter 9) can cause excessive sleepiness, a change of personality, adverse effects on social life and performance at work, and intel-lectual deterioration, sometimes to the extent that dementia is suspected.

Only a small minority of people with OSA go to see their doctor, probably because they do not realize that the cause of their problems is the often severe disruption of their sleep caused by this sleep disorder. Even those who have visited their doctor may well have been treated initially for the possible complications of their OSA (such as high blood pressure) before the eventual diagnosis of their sleep disorder is made. Clearly, correct recognition of this treatable condition is essential.

The same is true of children with OSA, which at this age is usually caused by enlarged tonsils and adenoids, the removal of which will generally improve daytime behaviour and learning difficulties that otherwise are likely to be attributed to the more usual psychological causes of these problems.

## Narcolepsy

Narcolepsy (see Chapter 9) is another, specific example of how sleepiness can be misinterpreted. Adults with this condition may be thought to be neurotic or to have a personality disorder or some other form of psychiatric disturbance.

When (as is usual) cataplexy is also present, there is even more scope for such mistakes. This part of the narcolepsy syndrome may be seen as fainting, epilepsy, or even attention-seeking behaviour. Often, many years elapse before narcolepsy is correctly diagnosed. In the meantime, sufferers usually receive all manner of inappropriate treatments or advice. It is quite possible that some cases of narcolepsy are never correctly recognized.

## Other sleep-related conditions

A number of other sleep-related conditions, although individually not particularly common, are also often not correctly recognized, with potentially serious consequences.

The particularly severe and episodic sleepiness in Kleine–Levin syndrome (see Chapter 9), often associated with strange and out-of-character behaviour when the person is awake, understandably causes confusion in the minds of those who are unfamiliar with the condition. Some people with this disorder are initially thought to have a serious brain disease, drug abuse problems, or a psychiatric illness.

Similarly, the violent behaviour at night displayed by some people with rapid eye movement (REM) sleep behaviour disorder (see Chapter 10), when acting out their dreams, is likely to be misconstrued, especially if the bed partner is attacked.

The form of sleep-related epilepsy known as 'nocturnal frontal lobe epilepsy' (see Chapter 10) also often involves seizures that include dramatic movements and noises. As these episodes are most unlike other types of epileptic seizures, it may be thought that the condition is not epilepsy at all but something quite different, such as a psychiatric disorder or pretending to have epilepsy.

## Overview

In considering all of these possible ways in which sleep disorders might not be recognized, it is, of course, important to realize that it is possible for someone to have both a sleep disorder and one or more other conditions of a different nature. This makes it all the more important (as described towards the beginning of this book) that both psychological and physical complaints, and their causes, are assessed thoroughly by someone familiar with the range of possible explanations, including a sleep disorder. Without this, there is a serious risk that a wrong conclusion will be reached, perhaps causing unnecessary concern, but also denying you the correct and effective treatment for your sleep disturbance.

To this extent, a sound knowledge of sleep disorders can be considered essential for all doctors, whether they work in general practice or—in view of the many ways in which sleep disorders can affect you—in medical and psychiatric specialties. The same is true for other healthcare professionals.

# 13

# Getting help with your sleep problem

## → Key points

◆ The help needed for your sleep problem, and who might provide it, depends on how severe and complicated the problem seems to be.

◆ Initially, self-help should be tried, i.e. good sleep hygiene (rather than self-medication).

◆ If the problem persists or is particularly worrying, consult your GP, who will, if necessary, refer you to a hospital specialist to assess your physical or psychological condition in more detail.

◆ Alternatively, your GP might feel that it is best to refer you directly to a sleep disorders clinic for a more detailed investigation and advice about treatment.

◆ A correct diagnosis should lead to specific treatment, which should be effective if carried out properly.

## ✖ Myth versus fact

✖ **Myth**: If you have a sleep problem, you can't do much about it except hope that it will go away.

❗ **Fact**: This is definitely not so. Much has been discovered about the prevention and treatment of the many types of sleep disorder. It is important to get help with your sleep problem because the consequences of not doing so can be serious.

# The importance of sleeping well

Satisfactory sleep is very important for various aspects of living, and for general health and well-being. Many of us may know that we have a sleep problem, but we might not always be fully aware of its possible consequences.

You may overlook the fact that your sleep is unsatisfactory and that it is likely to be at least partly responsible for making you feel below your best and unable to function properly during the day. It is important, therefore, to consider whether you, or any members of your family (or even friends), are showing the signs of unsatisfactory sleep described in Chapter 5.

# Helping yourself

If you suffer from insomnia and (possibly as a result) you are very sleepy during the day or affected in other ways, rather than treating yourself with over-the-counter products from the chemist or health food shop, see if you find it more helpful to try and improve your sleep hygiene (see Chapter 8). This may be all that is needed.

Remember that occasionally not sleeping well for a short time is common and is not a cause for concern. Parts of this book suggest additional ways in which you can at least make a start on helping yourself with other sleep issues such as jet lag, shift work, or driving problems, as well as having to care for others with conditions that disturb their sleep and, as a result, your own.

# Professional help

If your insomnia or excessive sleepiness persists, if you have frequent or worrying disturbances of your sleep, or if you have more than one type of sleep problem, you should seek professional advice. It has to be said that there is room for improvement in the training that professionals receive about sleep disorders, but the situation is slowly getting better, with more people taking an interest in the subject.

### Your family doctor

Your family doctor will at least be able to make a start in assessing your type of sleep problem and its cause, and may be able to suggest appropriate treatment for some conditions. Health visitors should be able to help with sleep problems in young children, who often disturb their parents' sleep.

## Specialist referral

Depending on the nature of your sleep problem, it may be advisable for you to be referred to a specialist in one or another branch of medicine. For example, you might see a specialist in respiratory medicine if your sleep is disturbed by a breathing difficulty. Referral to a psychiatrist is appropriate if the underlying problem seems to be depression or some other kind of long-standing psychological upset.

## Sleep disorders clinics

If the explanation for your sleep problem remains unclear, or seems particularly complicated or difficult to treat, you may need to be seen in a sleep disorders clinic. There are an increasing number of these in NHS hospitals (although many of them have a special interest only in problems of snoring and obstructive sleep apnoea in adults). Patients can sometimes be seen privately by staff working in some of these clinics. Alternatively, there are some exclusively private sleep disorders services.

A list of sleep disorders clinics, published by the British Sleep Society (see Useful addresses in the Appendix), can be requested by your GP to help decide where you can be referred.

The exact nature of the sleep problem, and its underlying cause, provide the basis on which choice of treatment depends, but adequate enquiries take time. They cannot be short-circuited without risking a superficial view of the problem, which is likely to result in inappropriate treatment or advice. Sometimes, more detailed information is needed before a diagnosis can be made, such as sleep recordings in hospital (see Chapter 6). Assessing the need for this, and carrying out the recordings, requires specialist advice and expertise.

If you are referred to a sleep disorders clinic, deciding on the specific treatment for your sleep disorder and supervising it is usually best done by the clinic staff. This might be a doctor or a psychologist, depending on the type of treatment. Your GP will usually be responsible for actually prescribing medication, if that is what is needed. You should then be followed up by your GP or the sleep clinic to see if the advice and treatment have been effective. If treatment is based on a careful analysis of the cause of your sleep problem, it can be expected to be effective in most cases when carried out under proper supervision.

Sleeping better can lead to significant improvements, not only in your own quality of life and prospects, but also in those of others affected by your sleep disorder.

# Appendix

## Useful addresses

British Sleep Society
PO Box 247
Colne
Huntington PE28 3UZ
Website: http://www.sleeping.org.uk

British Snoring and Sleep Apnoea Association
Castle Court
41 London Road
Reigate RH2 9RJ
Website: http://www.britishsnoring.co.uk

Narcolepsy Association UK (UKAN)
PO Box 13842
Penicuik EH26 8WX
Website: http://narcolepsy.org.uk/

## Sources of further information

### Non-technical

Stores, G. (2009) *Sleep Problems in Children and Adolescents: The Facts.* Oxford:
Oxford University Press.

### Technical

Kryger, M.H., Roth, T. & Dement, W.C. (eds) (2005) *Principles and Practice of
Sleep Medicine,* 4th edn. Philadephia: Elsevier Saunders. (A major textbook on
adult sleep and its disorders.)

Stores, G. (2001) *A Clinical Guide to Sleep and its Disorders in Children and Adolescents*. Cambridge: Cambridge University Press. (A textbook on sleep disorders from infancy to adolescence.)

American Academy of Sleep Medicine (2005) *International Classification of Sleep Disorders*, 2nd edition: *Diagnostic and Coding Manual*. Westchester, IL: American Academy of Sleep Medicine. (A systematic account of all officially recognized sleep disorders.)

# Glossary

The following are some of the technical terms used in this book.

**Active sleep:** equivalent in infants to REM sleep in subsequent development.

**Actometer (actigraph):** a wristwatch-like device that measures body movements to help distinguish between periods of sleep and wakefulness.

**Advanced sleep phase:** shift of the period of sleep to earlier than previously in the 24-hour sleep–wake cycle.

**Audio-visual recordings:** mainly recordings (including home video recordings by parents) to show a person's condition overnight. Can be particularly valuable in describing parasomnias and in obstructive sleep apnoea.

**Apnoea:** interruption of breathing (technically for a minimum of about 10 seconds).

**Arousal disorders or partial arousal disorders:** sleep disorders (confusional arousals, sleepwalking, and sleep terrors) that emerge abruptly from deep NREM sleep.

**Cataplexy:** sudden weakness provoked by strong emotions such as laughter, surprise, fear, or anger. Can cause a collapse or localized weakness lasting from a few seconds to minutes without loss of consciousness and with prompt recovery.

**Cerebrospinal fluid:** fluid within and surrounding the brain and spinal cord.

**Chronic fatigue syndrome (CFS), also known as myalgic encephalomyelitis (ME):** persistent or episodic fatigue and muscle pain of uncertain cause that does not lessen with sleep or rest.

**Chronotherapy:** treatment of sleep–wake cycle disorders by resetting the body clock.

**Chronotype:** whether you are alert and active mainly early in the day ('morningness' or 'lark' chronotype) or mainly late in the day ('eveningness' or 'owl' chronotype). Most people are neither one nor the other ('indifferent' chronotype).

**Circadian body clock:** system located in the suprachiasmatic nuclei in the depths of the brain, which, in conjunction with input from the eyes about light levels and output from the pineal gland of melatonin, determines the 24-hour sleep–wake rhythm.

**Circadian rhythm:** rhythm that occurs about once every 24 hours. Includes the sleep–wake cycle, which is normally tied to the 24-hour night–day cycle.

**Conditioned insomnia:** difficulty sleeping, the original cause of which no longer operates but which has led to habitual insomnia by association.

**Continuous positive airway pressure (CPAP):** device that delivers a stream of compressed air through a mask, keeping the upper airway open and preventing obstruction to breathing during sleep. An effective treatment for obstructive sleep apnoea.

**Delayed sleep phase:** shift of the sleep phase to later than previously in the 24-hour sleep–wake cycle.

**Desynchronization:** when things occur at unrelated times, as in sleep–wake cycle disorders where your sleep phase is out of time with your body temperature.

**Early morning waking:** in general, waking up before about 5 a.m. and not being able to go back to sleep.

**Electroencephalogram (EEG):** recording of the electrical activity of the brain by means of electrodes placed on the scalp. Combined with an electro-myogram and electro-oculogram, an EEG allows scoring of the sleep stages and wakefulness.

**Electromyogram:** recording of the electrical activity of muscles.

**Electro-oculogram:** recording of eye movements by means of electrodes placed on the face.

**Entrainment:** process by which your sleep–wake rhythm becomes linked to the 24-hour night–day cycle.

**Excessive (daytime) sleepiness or hypersomnia:** an increased tendency or need to fall asleep because of a sleep disorder.

**Fatigue:** lack of energy. Not necessarily associated with an increased tendency to fall asleep.

**Forbidden zone:** period of maximal alertness later in the day before the onset of sleepiness.

**Fragmentation of sleep:** interrupted sleep either by waking up repeatedly or by nearly doing so ('poor-quality sleep').

**Hypnagogic hallucinations (or imagery):** vivid perceptual experiences involving various senses. Can be alarming. Not uncommon and usually unassociated with any illness or disorder, but can be part of the narcolepsy syndrome.

**Hypnogram:** diagram of the structure of overnight sleep showing the sequence of sleep stages and periods of waking.

**Hypnopompic hallucinations or imagery:** unusual perceptual experiences when waking up.

**Hypocretin (orexin):** neurotransmitter in the brain involved in the control of sleep. Low levels are seen in people with narcolepsy/cataplexy.

**Infradian rhythm:** recurrent periods each lasting longer than 24 hours.

**Insomnia:** difficulty getting to sleep or staying asleep. Sometimes also refers to unrefreshing sleep.

**Light box:** lamp producing intense artificial illumination to simulate sunlight. Used for seasonal affective disorder and some circadian sleep–wake cycle disorders.

**Long sleeper:** person who habitually sleeps longer than most other people but without having a sleep disorder, i.e. at the upper end of the normal range of sleep requirements.

**Melatonin:** hormone secreted by the pineal gland. Regulates various biological functions including timing of sleep. Suppressed by light; production is stimulated in darkness (the 'hormone of darkness').

**Multiple sleep latency test:** objective test of sleepiness in which the opportunity to fall asleep is given several times during the day at regular intervals.

**Nap:** short period of sleep taken during the day.

**Narcolepsy syndrome:** group of symptoms, arising largely from a disorder of REM sleep, mainly comprising abnormal sleepiness (including brief 'sleep attacks'), cataplexy, hypnagogic hallucinations, and sleep paralysis.

**Nightmare:** frightening dream, arising in REM sleep (and therefore usually late in the night) that causes you to wake up.

**Non-rapid eye movement (NREM) sleep:** one of the two basic types of sleep, distinct from rapid eye movement (REM) sleep. Divided into four stages of increasing depth of sleep.

**Onset insomnia:** difficulty getting to sleep.

**Parasomnia:** episode of unusual behaviour or strange experience related to sleep.

**Parasomnia overlap disorder:** combination of arousal disorder and REM sleep behaviour disorder.

**Periodic limb movements in sleep (PLMS):** repetitive, brief, rapid flexion movements, mainly in the legs, during sleep.

**Pineal gland:** small gland in the centre of the brain that produces melatonin.

**Polysomnography (PSG):** continuous recording of sleep by means of an electroencephalogram, electromyogram, and electro-oculogram with the possible addition of breathing or other physiological measures depending on the nature of the sleep problem.

**Primary insomnia:** insomnia not caused by a mental or medical condition, drug, or other substance use or abuse, or by environmental factors.

**Quiet sleep:** the equivalent in infants of NREM sleep later in development.

**Rapid eye movement (REM) sleep:** type of sleep with the highest brain activity. Also known as 'dreaming sleep' because most dreaming occurs in it and 'paradoxical sleep' because, although brain activity is high, skeletal muscles are effectively paralysed.

**Seasonal affective disorder (SAD):** daytime fatigue and sleepiness, poor concentration, and increased appetite and weight gain, mainly in the winter months.

**Short sleeper:** person who habitually sleeps less than most other people but without having a sleep disorder, i.e. at the lower end of the normal range of sleep requirements.

**Sleep diary:** daily written record of a person's sleep–wake pattern and related events.

**Sleep disorder:** underlying condition causing a sleep problem.

**Sleep drive:** the extent to which we feel the need to sleep.

**Sleep drunkenness:** prolonged drowsiness, unsteadiness, and confusion after waking, despite having slept soundly.

**Sleep efficiency:** proportion of time in bed that a person actually sleeps.

**Sleep hygiene:** ways of improving sleep or preventing poor sleep.

**Sleep inertia:** a feeling of grogginess on waking up, especially from deep (slow-wave) sleep.

**Sleep maintenance insomnia:** waking repeatedly in the night.

**Sleep paralysis:** the brief inability to move or speak when falling asleep or waking up. May be accompanied by a feeling of being unable to breathe. Sometimes accompanied by hypnagogic hallucinations. Often an isolated experience, but can be part of the narcolepsy syndrome.

**Sleep phase:** period of sleep related to clock time.

**Sleep problem:** complaint of disturbed or abnormal sleep.

**Sleep start:** sudden brief movement or sensory experience when going off to sleep.

**Sleep–wake cycle:** alternation of sleep and wakefulness in each 24-hour period.

**Slow-wave sleep (SWS):** combination of stages 3 and 4 of NREM sleep, the deepest parts of sleep. Also called 'delta sleep' referring to the large slow (delta) waves that predominate.

**Snoring:** noise (which can be considerable) produced by a large intake of breath at the end of an apnoea. Caused by vibration of the soft palate and nearby structures.

**Suprachiasmatic nuclei:** groups of nerve cells located deep in the brain that control various bodily functions over each 24-hour period, including the sleep–wake rhythm.

**Ultradian rhythm:** recurrent period lasting less than 24 hours.

**Wind-down period:** gradually relaxing activities as bedtime approaches.

**Zeitgeber:** cue that informs the brain whether it is day or night, thus indicating when it is time to be awake or to sleep.

# Index